First, Do No Harm

Interpretive Studies in Healthcare and the Human Sciences

VOLUME 1

First, Do No Harm

Power, Oppression, and Violence in Healthcare

Nancy Diekelmann
Volume Editor

THE UNIVERSITY OF WISCONSIN PRESS

The University of Wisconsin Press
1930 Monroe Street
Madison, Wisconsin 53711

www.wisc.edu/wisconsinpress/

3 Henrietta Street
London WC2E 8LU, England

Library of Congress Cataloging-in-Publication Data

First, do no harm : power, oppression, and violence in healthcare / Nancy L. Diekelmann,
volume editor.
    p. ; cm. — (Interpretive studies in healthcare and the human sciences ; v. 1)
Includes bibliographical references and index.
  ISBN 0-299-17780-7 (cloth : alk. paper) — ISBN 0-299-17784-X (paper : alk. paper)
  1. Medical personnel and patient.   2. Quality of life.   3. Patients—Legal status, laws, etc.
4. Violence in hospitals.   5. Oppression (Psychology)
  [DNLM: 1. Professional-Patient Relations.   2. Delivery of Health Care.   3. Power
(Psychology)   4. Quality of Life.   5. Violence. WX 160 F527 2002]   I. Title: Power,
oppression, and violence in healthcare.   II. Diekelmann, Nancy L.   III. Series.
  R727.3 .F53 2002
  610.69′6—dc21

                                                              2001006771

To John Diekelmann and Jay Ironside, partners and soul mates, who never wavered in their love and encouragement

*In the midst of the constant noise of our modern world,
we need to create sufficient silence to hear ourselves
and others.*

James J. Fletcher, Mary Cipriano Silva, and Jeanne M. Sorrell,
"Harming Patients in the Name of Quality of Life"

Contents

Acknowledgments

Over the past 10 years, scholars from around the world have gathered at the University of Wisconsin–Madison Nursing Institutes for Heideggerian Hermeneutical Studies to examine hermeneutical methods and the interpretive phenomenology that underpins these approaches. The need for a book series arose when it became apparent that the contributions, richness, and complexity of interpretive studies in healthcare and the human sciences could not be shared within the traditional journal article page restrictions and format. Dedication to the timely publication of interpretive studies that would create converging conversation on a theme became the common vision. We are especially grateful to all the participants of the hermeneutical institutes for their inspiration, support, and encouragement, as this vision became a reality.

The members of the editorial board—David Allen, Michael Andrew, Patricia Benner, Karin Dahlberg, Daniel W. Jones, Kathryn Hopkins Kavanagh, Fred Kersten, Birgit Negussie, and Thomas Sheehan—were central in shaping the book series and have provided expert consultation along the way. They have kept the bar of scholarship high. We owe special thanks to Nadine Cross, Kathryn Kavanagh, Marie Hayden-Miles, and Jeanne Sorrell, who never failed to come through for us on a moment's notice. These women created a place in their scholarship to accompany us through the many complexities of getting a new book series off the ground. Most important however, is that they have consistently supported and encouraged us with their wisdom, insight, and friendship. We are forever indebted.

Our heartfelt thanks and appreciation go to John Diekelmann, Fred

Kersten, and Tom Sheehan. These philosophical thinkers have given unselfishly of their expertise in interpretive phenomenology to guide the development of a rigorous interpretive tradition in the health and human sciences. Their questions, comments, and insights have consistently challenged, extended, and enhanced this scholarship. They have supported this project in many practical ways, but it is their unwavering belief in the importance of this work that means the most.

We would also like to thank Cathy Andrews, Lea Rae Galarowicz, Cathy Nosek, Martha Scheckel, and Tricia Young for the many ways they contributed to this project. They have been our partners in this project and in the annual institutes. Their willingness to take up any task to see that this scholarship moves forward has been remarkable.

We are grateful to Julie Boddy, Margaret Douglas, Claire Draucker, James Fletcher, Frances Henderson, Joanne Hessmiller, Mary LeBold, Birgit Negussie, Mary Silva, Sheri Sims, Liz Smythe, Melinda Swenson, and Chris Tanner for their strong support of this project and for their work toward ensuring that international perspectives were safeguarded. Their enthusiasm and encouragement has sustained us throughout this endeavor. Similarly, we are grateful to Gloria Barsness, Morgan Harlow, Yvette La Pierre, and Patricia Wilcox for their technical and editorial expertise. They have been instrumental in bringing this text to print and in providing the connections between and among editors and contributors working at a distance. Sue Breckenridge has been the production guide for this project, and her timely commentary has made all the difference. Without the diligent commitment of Robert Mandel, director of the University of Wisconsin Press, and Stephen Salemson, associate director, this book series would not have been possible. As forward-thinking scholars they recognized the endowment this series creates toward moving to re-form contemporary healthcare and overcoming extant challenges in the human sciences.

Last but not least, we would like to thank Vivian Littlefield, Dean Emerita, and Katharyn May, Dean of the School of Nursing at the University of Wisconsin–Madison, for creating a place for interpretive scholars to gather each year. In the midst of multiple economic challenges across higher education, their commitment to and support of scholarship in the human sciences that creates a neoteric future for healthcare has been steadfast and truly noteworthy.

Nancy L. Diekelmann and Pamela M. Ironside

Foreword

Kathryn Hopkins Kavanagh

Occasionally an opportunity reveals itself that opens new ways for exploring commonplace things that *matter.* This volume represents one of those rare chances to deviate from acedian paths to explore new philosophies in monographic depth. The first of a neoteric (even revolutionary) book series, *Interpretive Studies in Healthcare and the Human Sciences,* this inaugural volume embodies new perspectives and vanguard research of violence, power, and oppression in the context of contemporary healthcare. The chapters reflect solid, expert research and authorship, as well as the editors' premium standards. Given the unsettling and unintended, albeit often rather mysterious (or at least not well understood), meanings of health and healthcare, the selections contribute a greatly needed, even essential, view of experiences today. I look forward to using these interpretive studies in teaching medical anthropology. I know that other educators will find them equally valuable in a variety of courses as the volume opens deep conversations among differing ways of thinking and behaving. The *real life* personal phenomena reflected in these chapters afford glimpses of praxis at its most elucidating: the confluence of research, theory, and practice under a critical gaze. And best of all, the reading is good!

First, Do No Harm: Power, Oppression, and Violence in Healthcare and the Human Sciences addresses vulnerability in the context of healthcare. In addressing such potent experiences as violence and vulnerability, power and oppression, the volume mindfully avoids imposing the conceptual burdens of restrictive definitions. Instead, it summons experiential ownership of authentic but diverse perceptions, reflections, and realities relating to those themes. The volume is strategic, in light of the megatrend toward new political identities and special interests. Refreshingly and unpretentiously, the studies yield far more questions than answers.

Vulnerability is about some individuals and groups becoming victims, and others survivors. It is more than multidisciplinary—not peculiar to professional disciplines or academia—but central to living. Dissatisfied with being herded along in systems rife with problems, people are seeking healthful and healing alternatives. The search is so integral a part of contemporary culture that its discussion crosses every perspective. Curative medicine, although still powerful, is having its taken-for-granted authority (and certainly the sporadic innuendoes of omnipotence, omniscience, and omnipresence that have historically accompanied the paradigm) *questioned*. Such transformation is embedded in and confounded by cultural customs and social expectations. Making these cultural customs and social expectations explicit is essential to a society ready to move beyond consumer information, which, by leaving the onus on the consumer, too often lends itself to increasing vulnerability.

The quest is for cultural transformation rooted in the conviction that vulnerability and oppression are real and unjust, while meaningful advocacy is and must be cost effective in *all* ways, including productivity and quality of life. The ideas expressed in these chapters are cutting edge, exciting (although at times bewildering), and ready for readers to take them in myriad academic and professional directions. The need is documented, the potential for change genuine. We are a long way from having adequate positivistic evidence to support many issues as they are played out in real life. The groundwork for useful understanding has to come through interpretive scholarship to be substantive and convincing. But to be valuable, it also requires the authority of rigorous scholarly inquiry; it cannot be merely impressionistic. As many aspects of healthcare become increasingly technical, and surely the complexity of technology and subsequent fragmentation of knowledge and practice reinforce this, we intensely need the views of scholars who can envision the larger picture, in addition to erudite articulations of how the quotidian thrust of fragmenting systems of knowledge may be experienced in their application.

In sum, the new book series and this first volume will make significant contributions to understanding sociocultural as well as personal and medical constructions of the body and being in health and illness. I question whether anyone other than Nancy Diekelmann could muster the support to bring such a series to life and to sustain it, but she has, can, and will. Only such an accomplished and catalytic scholar could elicit and oversee such quality studies. This volume is historic in its message. It is a call to scholars, researchers, students, and citizens to participate in new conversations. Power, oppression, and violence, as their experience is reflected in these studies, call forth new understandings. I trust that future volumes will have more contributions from disciplines not yet represented and be even more international. People concerned with interpretive issues in healthcare are out there—more of them all the time—and many of them seek the level of intellectual challenge and stimulation found in *Interpretive Studies in Healthcare and the Human Sciences*.

Introduction

Nancy L. Diekelmann

Healthcare around the world has reached a perilous state. Issues emanating from the explosion of biomedical technologies and the industrialization and depersonalization of healthcare are no longer merely the concerns of practitioners; everyone is noticing. Enabled by access to the latest biomedical information, constituents are increasingly challenging the traditional power structure of contemporary healthcare systems and raising substantive concerns about oppression and violence embedded in issues such as access to and quality of healthcare. No longer are the machinations of contemporary healthcare delivery systems (which have silently moved away from interaction and collaboration with the person as patient to the mere observation of patients as sources of data to be collected and analyzed) conferred upon silent, passive, uninformed subjects. The fervor of the discourse challenging the current healthcare system and practices around the world reveals that power, oppression, and violence can no longer be considered simply issues that healthcare practitioners address (or treat) and that human scientists investigate. Rather, the studies in this book explicate how power, oppression, and violence are implicitly embedded in the very practices directed toward their alleviation. This volume brings the dynamics of the meanings of violence and its significance into active discourse.

This book is a gathering of many voices. Practitioners, students, teachers, scholars, and citizens from around the world and from across disciplines join in converging conversations to explore multiple perspectives and contexts. Such multifaceted conversations draw the reader into pondering the richness and complexity as well as the dangers of current healthcare practices. Without resorting to simplistic explanations or arguments, power, violence, and oppression are not objectified as characteristics of a particular, although substantive, problem to be solved. The conversations in this book resist the familiar exposé or overdramatization positing political statements of reform. Rather, these studies reveal how power, violence, and oppression accompany, although inadvertently, some of the "best practices" of healthcare. The narratives in these studies illustrate how "good folks," professionals with the best of intentions, perpetrate violence while attempting to provide the best, most holistic care possible. In this way, the studies in this volume are unsettling for healthcare professionals because it is much easier to see each of these issues as a problem of the "other." These studies uncompromisingly show how power, violence, and oppression are close at hand.

The authors in this volume describe how power, oppression, and violence are experienced as people struggle to sustain meaningful lives and relationships while receiving healthcare. Extending from birthing to end-of-life decisions, the authors explore the provision of state-of-the-art healthcare as well as the withholding of even basic care. The interpretive studies in this book do not avoid profoundly questioning extant knowledge and practice issues that reproduce the assumption that biomedical–technological solutions are the only possibility for the reform or improvement of healthcare. Each author illuminates new possibilities for recognizing, understanding, and overcoming oppressive power practices and violence in ways that are often at hand and already present in contemporary healthcare.

This book is also the gathering of diverse interpretive methodologies and traditions around a common interest: power, violence, and oppression in healthcare and human sciences. Moving beyond methodological nationalism in scholarship, this volume reflects how gathering interpretive methodologies can not only enhance and extend what is known about violence, power, and oppression but also can raise complex, multifaceted questions to elicit and encourage continued thought and inquiry. Interpretive studies challenge and extend scientific scholarship by prying open to questioning the underlying presuppositions of the universality that forms the basis for science. Thought of in this way, these interpretive studies are a beginning—a questioning that gathers practitioners, students, teachers, scholars, and citizens into persistent thinking and conversation around complex contemporary issues.

The new book series *Interpretive Studies in Healthcare and the Human Sciences* creates an ongoing forum for practitioners, students, teachers, scholars, and citizens to participate in international, interdisciplinary interpretive conversations about selected contemporary issues in healthcare and the human sciences. In each volume, scholars employing diverse interpretive approaches (specifically, interpretive phenomenology, ethnography, grounded theory, narrative analysis, symbolic interactionism, critical social theory, feminist theory, and postmodern discourses) explore contemporary issues, complex questions, and current practices to both contribute to and challenge extant knowledge and understanding in the health sciences. The new book series also creates a place for interpretive studies to be presented in detail so that the richness and depth of the explication as well as the theoretical and philosophical underpinnings of the methodology can be fully described. In this way, experienced interpretive scholars and students of interpretive approaches, those practicing from within and from outside the interpretive paradigms, and those within and outside the healthcare disciplines can join ongoing dialogues. Through reflective thinking that responds to contemporary issues from a variety of perspectives, neoteric approaches to healthcare are explored.

This volume, the first in the series *Interpretive Studies in Healthcare and the Human Sciences,* heralds a movement to overcome power, violence, and oppression in the health and human sciences by gathering substantive international scholarship into converging conversations. The chapters in this volume exquisitely reveal what has been dismissed, ignored, or simply forgotten in contemporary healthcare research and practice, illuminating once again that issues of power, violence, and oppression know no borders.

First, Do No Harm

1

Harming Patients in the Name of Quality of Life

*James J. Fletcher, Mary Cipriano Silva,
and Jeanne M. Sorrell*

The term *quality of life* is used widely in healthcare literature, yet there is surprisingly little agreement as to its precise meaning (Goodinson & Singleton, 1989). In this chapter we will undertake an examination of the meanings and uses of this concept, especially as the concept is appealed to in making clinical decisions about treatment for people experiencing dementia. Decision making is evidence of power. Oppression is associated with abusive or unreasonable use of decision making. Usually an unequal power balance exists between the oppressor and the oppressed, which results in the oppressed feeling diminished as a valued person. Too often, with good intentions but limited insight, healthcare professionals oppress those entrusted to their care, thus harming them in the name of quality of life. It is our contention that quality of life as it has been used contributes to oppressive behavior and is based on an incomplete model of medicine that is particularly inappropriate for fragile populations suffering from the isolating and discontinuous experiences of dementia. The appeal to a quality-of-life standard in making clinical decisions is ostensibly an attempt to ensure objectivity whether the decision is to initiate, withhold, or withdraw therapeutic interventions, including life-sustaining treatment. Our research indicates that the sought after objectivity is elusive at best. We contend that the usual bases for reaching judgments about quality of life fail to take into consid-

3

eration important elements essential to determining the appropriate clinical interventions for those experiencing dementia.

In part 1 of this chapter we examine the concept of quality of life, distinguishing between descriptive, evaluative, and normative meanings of the term and their applications in clinical decision making. We then describe a model of medicine that grounds the appeal to quality-of-life considerations and show how this model leads to a distortion not only of clinical decision making but also of our understanding of the phenomenon of aging. We conclude part 1 by endorsing an alternative model, which we then employ in the second and third parts of the chapter to address dementia and the relationship of spirituality to personhood, quality of life, and violence. In part 2 of this chapter we discuss the concept of life interpretation in the context of illness. Excerpts from a phenomenological study of ethical concerns of patients and carers living with Alzheimer's Disease are used to focus on three concepts: (1) the power of the healthcare system; (2) the power of the healthcare provider; and (3) life narratives of persons with Alzheimer's Disease. In part 3 we focus on personhood, spirituality, and quality of life for persons with dementia. While some may equate spirituality and religiosity, we do not. Following Hiatt (1986), we view the spiritual as "that part of the person concerned with meaning . . . and the ultimate significance of things" (p. 737). Given the fragmentation that generally accompanies dementia, it is especially important to recognize that the spiritual dimension plays an integrative function for individuals (Hiatt, 1986). Finally, we discuss two definitions of spirituality, and we argue that attention to spirituality can, especially in its integrative function, enhance the quality of life for persons with dementia.

Part 1. Quality of Life and Medical Decision Making

The Meaning of Quality of Life

The claim that persons are to be valued and, therefore, that humans should be protected and their lives maintained has been a constant throughout the history of Western ethics. With attention to hygiene and sterile conditions in medical practice, the development of antibiotics to combat infectious diseases, and the more recent developments of medical technology, the incidence of chronic and disabling diseases like cancer and cardiovascular disease has increased dramatically (Musschenga,

1997). The development of technology has been especially problematic because, for example, the use of mechanical ventilators can allow individuals to be kept "alive" long past the time that their bodies could sustain life on their own. Collectively, these circumstances led clinicians and family members to question the wisdom of intervening to resuscitate or maintain a life that cannot be restored to a healthy condition and which would be heavily burdened from the side effects of the intervention. Thus, starting in the 1950s and especially in the 1970s the use of the term quality of life became popular as a way of questioning the appropriateness of certain interventions (Musschenga, 1997; Reich, 1978).

For some the term quality of life is used in contrast to the term *sanctity of life* to express contrasting attitudes toward maintaining biological life (Reich, 1978). Sanctity of life is said to express an absolutist position on preserving physical life, advocating mere survival and refusing to consider the quality of that life. In contrast, those advocating a quality-of-life ethics deny that human life has a sacred value and must be maintained despite the condition of that life (Fletcher, 1975). Those who advocate a sanctity-of-life ethic generally follow a deontological theory holding that a life has value in itself, irrespective of its condition. Quality-of-life advocates tend to be consequentialists in their approach to ethics, arguing that the maintenance and protection of a human life is not an overriding obligation in the absence of certain minimum qualities or characteristics (Reich, 1978). Carlberg (1998) argues that sanctity of life does not require one to be indifferent to the conditions under which a life is lived. He states:

As long as biological human life is not disassociated from personal human life, there need not be a divide separating the sanctity and the quality of life. It is quite legitimate for physicians and bioethicists to specify the attributes that would normally constitute human life as a good worth sustaining—and hence to delineate the limits of our positive obligations to preserve it—without drawing the conceptually erroneous conclusion that death is, in certain circumstances, better than life, or for that matter, that life is always better than death. (pp. 195–196)

So, according to Carlberg, it is legitimate to raise questions about the quality of life in making clinical decisions. The problem, of course, is in reaching agreement on "the attributes that would normally constitute human life as a good worth sustaining." While deciding this is a task beyond the scope of our chapter, we begin our study by taking a closer look at the meaning of quality of life and the approach that some have taken to articulate a minimum standard for a life worth sustaining.

Quality of life has been used with *descriptive, evaluative,* and *normative* meanings in healthcare literature (Aiken, 1982; Musschenga, 1997; Reich, 1978; Walter, 1995). As a descriptive concept, quality of life designates certain properties that can be used for comparison purposes to measure the differences among people or social groups. This use of the term most often occurs in the social sciences. In a recent review of quality-of-life instruments used in clinical settings, Gill and Feinstein (1994) identify approximately 150 instruments used in 75 articles that they reviewed. Significantly, most of these instruments focus on a set of indicators that can be used to measure an individual's ability to function "normally" and independently in some fashion or other; we will return to this point later because of its implications for interpreting modern medicine's approach to health.

When quality of life is used in an evaluative sense, it "indicates that some value or worth is attached either to a characteristic of a person (for example, capacity to choose) or to a type of life that is lived (for example, free of pain and handicap)" (Walter, 1995, p. 1353). In the evaluative sense, quality of life means that a feature or set of features is desirable and ought to be appreciated or even to be considered sacred. Frequently, the designated feature is said to be a necessary condition for humanhood or personhood. The literature exhibits a wide range of candidates for this designation, including: simple biological life (Walter, 1988), reason, cognitive functioning (Veatch, 1993), minimal independence (Shelp, 1986), and potential for human relationships (McCormick, 1974). Fletcher (1972, 1974) points to a set of "indicators of humanhood," prominent among which are self-awareness, concern for others, curiosity, and balancing rationality with feeling. It is not hard to conclude that individuals suffering advanced stages of dementia may have a difficult time meeting these standards of humanhood. Reich (1978) distinguishes the properties of humanhood from what he calls accessory qualities. The former are "those distinctively human qualities so valued that they are seen as necessary conditions for extending to humans possessing them the benefit of those norms that the human moral community offers for the preservation of life" (Reich, 1978, p. 834). In contrast, "accessory qualities are secondary or subordinate qualities that are regarded as criteria for either intensifying or diminishing the obligation to preserve life" (Reich, 1978, p. 834). In determining whether a valued characteristic or set of characteristics is present, clinicians might make use of one of the many instruments studied by Gill and Feinstein (1994) to determine a patient's status ranging from fully conscious without disabilities to unconscious or to judge the patient to be in a state ranging from no distress to severe distress. Among the accessory qualities that might be measured are the patient's awareness, mobility, physical activity, self-care, social relationships, and mood (Edgar, 1998).

We now consider the normative sense of quality of life. The normative meaning is most significant for bioethics because it provides moral reasons for clinical decisions to initiate, withhold, or withdraw treatment. In effect, quality of life is appealed to normatively when it is necessary to deal with conflict situations, especially "whether one ought to support and protect life on the basis of a perception of human qualities" (Reich, 1978, p. 831). As Walter (1995) notes:

Morally normative or prescriptive claims about a quality of life always involve a moral judgment on the valued quality and, by implication, a judgment on the life that possesses that quality. These . . . statements, then, not only presume that a quality—for example, cognitive ability—is valued, but they also entail judgments about whether, and under which conditions, one must or ought to protect and preserve a life that possesses the valued quality or qualities. (p. 1353)

Such judgments are frequently exercised in the form of an exclusionary judgment; that is, the quality-of-life criterion is a reason for excluding some from the moral community and, therefore, from the normal standards of treatment (Aiken, 1982). This can be illustrated by Reich's account of how McCormick's (1974) use of potentiality for human relationships functions normatively. Reich (1978) writes:

The humanhood quality or key criterion for determining whether there is a duty to preserve life is thus the *relational potential* of the individual. If this potentiality is absent or completely subordinated to the mere effort for survival, the individual may be allowed to die. (p. 835)

In using quality of life criteria to determine whether or not normal medical standards of treatment are either appropriate or required, there are two principal considerations. The first is whether the treatment will result in a minimal level of human functioning, taking pain and disability into consideration; the second involves whether the patient will succeed in achieving a minimum level of development (Musschenga, 1997). While the second consideration most often involves decisions about treating defective newborns, it is clear that the same type of quality of life is applicable to individuals experiencing severe dementia where the question is whether such individuals can maintain a sufficient level of development. It is here that we find considerable potential for oppressing such individuals.

Quality of Life Measurements

On what bases are quality-of-life judgments made? In the early 1970s, an effort was made to make such decisions objective by appealing to indicators that measure normal functioning and independence (Musschenga, 1997). This led to the development and use of a wide range of instruments such as the Karnofsky Performance Index (Karnofsky & Burchenal, 1949), the Spitzer Quality of Life Index (Spitzer, Dobson, Hall, Chesterman, & Levi, 1981), and others such as those considered by Gill and Feinstein (1994). In addition, during the 1980s social scientists began insisting on the importance of patient satisfaction as an important, subjective source of decisions about quality of life in determining the suitability of treatment options. A patient's limited ability to function may rule out a range of treatment options that might otherwise be a treatment of choice for a particular disease or condition. On the other hand, it is also important to determine a patient's overall level of satisfaction. In this regard, the force of the criteria depends on the individual's own judgment of what qualities, physical well-being, mental capacity, social relatedness, or spiritual satisfaction are required for continued existence. The importance of obtaining the patient's view of the quality of his or her life is underlined by the findings of Spitzer et al. (1981) that patients rate themselves higher in quality-of-life measures than do their physicians, and of Starr, Pearlman, and Uhlmann (1986) that physicians do not do well in anticipating whether their elderly patients will execute do not resuscitate (DNR) orders. Musschenga (1997) notes that quality-of-life research is:

only weakly linked to objective conditions, such as age, gender, income, conditions of living and also health, but highly to social ones, such as the availability of social support, and psychological ones, especially personality traits as feeling of competence, ego-strength, feeling of having control over one's life, maturity, optimism, etc. (p. 24)

Quality-of-life judgments tend to be summative assessments of the conditions of lives. They can be made either at a personal or at a societal level. In the former case they represent either a degree of satisfaction with the circumstances of one's life based on self-perception (Young & Longman, 1983) or normative judgments about personhood that may impact clinical decisions concerning therapeutic interventions. Quality of life applied at the personal level is the primary sense in which we are using this term in our chapter. At the societal level, quality-of-life considerations are used in the calculation of what is called a *quality adjusted life year* (QALY). Since this term appears frequently in the literature, it is important to explain it and to differentiate it from quality-of-life judgments at the personal level.

Quality adjusted life years. QALY has become a generic term for a class of quality-of-life indicators (Edgar, 1998). However calculated, all QALYs are a "numerical description of the value that a medical procedure or service can provide to groups of patients with similar medical conditions" (LaPuma & Lawlor, 1990, p. 2917). QALYs function chiefly as tools of health economics (Edgar, 1998); as such they function at the macro level of decision making. QALYs are established by sampling large segments of the population to learn from their experiences of illness and disease the extent to which certain healthcare interventions cost-effectively produce benefits greater than the suffering that may accompany them. Since many chronic conditions are not curable, relative weight must be given to quality of life and duration of life (Goodinson & Singleton, 1989; Stoll, 1977). One way to determine QALYs is to ask segments of the population about their willingness to imaginatively "trade years of life for different presentations of quality of life. . . . QALYs 'discount' years of life saved by a healthcare intervention by how much patients' subjective well-being is diminished by comfort or distress" (LaPuma & Lawlor, p. 2917). Beginning with basic data on survival, the QALY measure does not treat all years of survival as equal in value; lower scores are assigned to any years spent in poor health (Edgar, 1998). Using such analyses, policy makers try to ensure that healthcare resources are used effectively and to make judgments about the rationing of healthcare. Such a procedure was used in Oregon to determine the application of Medicaid services. For our purposes it is important to recognize that QALYs are based on aggregate community preferences and that the process of clinical decision making is not part of the measures that constitute QALYs (LaPuma & Lawlor, 1990). Goodinson and Singleton (1989) point out that:

An assumption inherent in the concept of a QALY,[sic] is that it is appropriate to use the evaluations of 70 "healthy" respondents as though this yielded information which is universally applicable. This ignores the individual patient's own evaluation of life and undermines his autonomy. It is assumed that the evaluations incorporated in the concept of a QALY have objectivity and are thus universal for all subjects. (p. 336)

The attraction and widespread use of QALYs in healthcare economics reflect an assumption operating at all levels of healthcare, namely that introducing more subtle scientific measures and procedures can determine the right course of action in a more objective manner. It is part of a trend in modern medicine toward a scientific pursuit of certainty.

Quality of Life and the Biomedical Model of Medicine

Leplege and Hunt (1997) express concern about what they call the medical model approach to quality-of-life measurements. The medical model interpretation of quality of life places an overwhelming emphasis on function and interprets quality of life in terms of its components. They remark that:

The fact that the types of questionnaires currently used to measure quality of life place an overwhelming emphasis on functional capacity may be because of the dominance of the medical model stressing the ability to perform everyday tasks and fulfill occupational and social roles. (p. 48)

One consequence of this is that the meaning and importance that individuals give to these tasks and roles is discounted in deference to professional judgments (Hahn, 1995; Leplege & Hunt, 1997). Using the medical model to preserve professional judgments of quality of life clearly has implications for aging populations and those experiencing dementia. As Leplege and Hunt state, "to imply that physically disabled or elderly persons have a poorer quality of life than younger or able-bodied individuals is a reinforcement of stereotypes that underlie discriminatory practices" (p. 48). The potential for devaluing the elderly is increased under this interpretation. The more one is devalued, the more likely one may suffer violence and oppression.

The medical model to which they refer is an outgrowth of the success that Western medicine has achieved by its reliance on the scientific, experimental method. Medicine is both an art and a science, but, in its recent development, the art of medicine has been superceded by medicine as science. Inasmuch as medicine has associated itself with science, it has achieved the trust and acceptance of society (Estes & Binney, 1989). Among the marks of medicine as science are: objectivity, problem solving, reductionism, and precision. Stein (1990) relates this closely to American cultural values. He writes:

In the United States . . . disease conceptualization and treatment are embedded in the value system of self reliance, rugged individualism, independence, pragmatism, empiricism, atomism, privatism, emotional minimalism, and a mechanistic conception of the body and its "repair". . . . The biomedical conceptualization and treatment of disease have been welcomed and have successfully "diffused" in American culture precisely because they fit so well with the image of the self as a physical object that can be broken and fixed. (p. 21)

The dominance of this view of medicine is reflected in the recent attempts to approach critical and terminal care decisions in terms of judgments about medical futility (Keyserlingk, 1997).

Medicine and power. Medicine has always had a hierarchical structure, with the physician as the dominant figure and the source of most decisions about treatment. One must appreciate that the role of the physician is part of the culture of American medicine (Stein, 1990). Stein points out that, in addition to providing the knowledge and techniques required to fight disease, "the central task of medical education is the transformation of a lay or 'civilian' person into the role and status of a physician . . . [including] the creation of boundaries" (pp. 179–180). In an earlier, less complex time the relationship of the physician to the patient was usually based on long experience and intimate knowledge of both the patient's and the patient's family's health history. The close relationship, based on knowledge and trust, contributed to inappropriate paternalism by which the physician acted on behalf of the patient's welfare even if it was not what the patient wished. Recent attention to the autonomy of the patient in deciding the type and extent of treatment has resulted in a sharing of power not only with the patient but also with other healthcare professionals who have independent responsibility to act as the patient's advocate. Despite the importance of autonomy, the operative definitions of "health" and "wellness" rest largely in the determination of healthcare personnel (Hahn, 1995). Much of this is articulated in the quality-of-life instruments previously mentioned.

The success of modern scientific medicine has created a system that envelops and dominates patients and practitioners alike. Medicine, with its emphasis on technology, has succumbed to what Habermas (1984) calls the distortion of systematic rationalization. In place of individual consultation and intimate knowledge, there is an automated system of analysis coupled with a defined set of options. The systemization already initiated by the "technolization" of medicine has been accelerated by the introduction of managed care. Under the current rules, decisions about treatment may be made by individuals who have never communicated with the patient or may be subject to a predetermined set of options resulting from a QALY study, as in the case of the Oregon Medicaid protocol. In such instances, patients and healthcare professionals alike become subject to the demands of the system. Within systematic medicine success means cure, conquering disease, and restoring health (Hahn, 1995). But the key to the scientific model of medicine lies in the reductive approach it has taken to the problem of human illness. Consider the following observations by Cassell (1993):

The first [reductive] step [in the history of medicine] was reducing the problem of human illness—with all of its intricate physical, social, emotional, and cultural aspects—to the biological problem of disease. Diseases were initially defined as physical entities with unique anatomical (later biochemical) characteristics and unique causes. These two unique characteristics permitted precise definitions. Precise definitions . . . permitted the productive entrance of science into medicine. The second reductive step follows from the scientific investigation of diseases. Here the findings of science become the accepted picture of the disease, further oversimplifying the problem. The scientific discovery of the disease agent completes the simplification as the agent, for example, the tubercle bacillus, becomes the virtual equivalent of the disease, tuberculosis. (p. 33)

With illness reduced, scientifically, to disease, only scientifically trained individuals could really participate in the decision-making process, with the consequence that "meaningful" judgments on matters of health came to reflect primarily the healthcare professional's point of view.

The dominance of the reductionist view of medicine has been reinforced by the rapid development of medical technology. As Cassell (1993) writes, "Medical technology's form and character arise from medicine's focus on disease and pathophysiology as the arena in which the origins and solutions to human sickness are to be found" (p. 39). What is needed, Cassell contends, is a reorientation of medicine to the whole person and away from the focus on disease. A similar reduction has taken place in recent interpretations of aging, which Estes and Binney (1989) describe as the "biomedicalization of aging" (p. 587).

The medical model applied to aging. The biomedicalization of aging represents a restrictive analysis of the aging process that focuses almost exclusively on the biological and scientific aspects of aging such that the normal process of growing old is reconstructed as a medical problem. Estes and Binney (1989) explain:

The construction of aging as a medical problem focuses on the diseases of the elderly—their etiology, treatment, and management—from the perspective of the practice of medicine as defined by practitioners. This means that the medical model—with its emphasis on clinical phenomena—takes precedence over, and in many cases defines, the basic biological, social, and behavioral processes and problems of aging. (pp. 587–588)

Society has become convinced of the appropriateness of this approach to the problem of aging. While the biomedical model has succeeded in providing sophisticated diagnoses and therapeutic interventions for diseases associated with the elderly, the equation of old age with illness leads society to think of aging itself as a pathology and, hence, abnormal, resulting in decline, disability, degeneration, and death. Equating the physical condition of aging with illness also affects how the elderly view themselves and how they see their place in society (Estes, 1979). Eventually the elderly become convinced that they are ill and begin to exhibit the behavior associated with disease, including social withdrawal, reduction of activity, and increased dependency (Estes & Binney, 1989). And, as they point out, by placing the primary focus on disease, society has limited its consideration of larger social and environmental factors. Moreover, the culture of medicine, with its focus on success as cure, makes it very difficult to deal with chronic conditions. The frustration of practitioners is expressed in the following remarks by a family physician:

I like to do a lot of OB [obstetrics]. There's an end point, and you know you're done. The woman is pregnant, I deliver her baby, and that's a cure. You can see the results of your work, a finished product. I know they say now that pregnancy isn't a disease, but you know what I mean. I get the same feeling doing surgery, and I know that's the reason people go into surgery and OB. They want results. They want something to show for it when they're done. . . . It's so different treating chronic illness. You do your goal setting, but end up feeling like a failure because the patient isn't cured. (Stein, 1990, p. 30)

This passage demonstrates the extent to which the biomedical model is focused on the metaphor of disease. In such a culture, aging itself is sufficient to subject one to what Foucault (1973) has called the "clinical gaze," whereby individuals become equated with their conditions and reduced to physiological phenomena. We believe that the dominance of the biomedical model of aging is reflected in the stories related later in this chapter. One of the lessons of those stories is that viewing aging primarily as a medical problem makes it difficult to deal with the social, environmental, and economic dimensions of the aging experience that are so prominent in the narratives of both the elderly and their family members. Estes and Binney (1989) point out that the biomedical model has been unable

to address macrostructural problems implicated in the etiology of ill health. Medicine's response has been to focus attention on individual health behaviors and life-styles, making the individual responsible for illness. In contrast, social and behavioral sciences research and the success of the life-course perspective model point to the inadequacy of the biomedical model based on unicausal, homogenous, and inevitable biological processes. (p. 595)

We believe that the failure of the biomedical model is reflected in the practices that dominate care of the elderly in nursing homes, especially the tendency to medically manage behavior through the use of drugs. The major point we want to make is summarized in the following passage from Moody (1992):

The medical model constitutes a specific mode of interpreting human experience, including the experience of illness. It adopts an instrumental, rather than a hermeneutic view of experience. Specifically, the medical model entails a causal-reductive approach that excludes dimensions of meaning, above all the meaning of suffering. We can appreciate the significance of this point in thinking about medical views of the handicapped and the mentally retarded, who also constitute a class of patients with an incurable disorder. Where Dostoyevsky, for instance, could see in the retarded an echo of the Christian ideal—the "fool of God"—modern societies see only diminished capacity and the extinction of personhood. (p. 68)

A Phenomenological Alternative

A well-articulated alternative model for approaching the phenomenon of dementia is provided by Lyman (1998). Without denying the reality of physical decline that accompanies aging, Lyman rejects exclusive attention to the physical in favor of what she calls a "sociomedical model of disability" (p. 52). She begins by asking: "How do older people negotiate their social relationships and individual identities to incorporate the changes associated with chronic conditions?" (p. 49). The force of the change in models is immediately apparent because Lyman tells us that she is "interested in the viewpoint of older persons who live with the extremes of impairment, loss, and dependency, people with Alzheimer's Disease or other dementing illnesses" (p. 49). Starting with the viewpoints of older persons enables her to rethink the prevailing paradigm of dementia as "loss," particularly "loss of self" stemming from the physical deterioration of specific structures and regions of the brain.

To escape the limitations of the biomedical model, Lyman (1998) adopts a phenomenological perspective and turns to the elderly themselves so that her account can be based on their lived experiences. The contrast in the models is striking:

The explanation of troublesome behavior among people with dementia locates the biomedical model within the "medicalization of deviance" tradition: misbehavior represents individual pathology of somatic or organic etiology, to be diagnosed, treated and managed according to medical authority. . . . A phenomenological alternative to the biomedical model of dementia focuses on the "experience of illness," rather than "disease progression." This perspective emphasizes modifiable conditions that affect the illness experience, in contrast with the biomedical model's deterministic view, which attributes the individual's functioning and behavior problems to the neuropathology of dementia. (pp. 49–50)

Escaping the determinism of the biomedical model requires a change in language. Instead of *disease*, which denotes a healthcare professional's diagnosis of a bio-physiological condition, Lyman recommends that we speak of *illness*, which connotes a subjective, sociopsychological experience perceived by an individual. Additional changes in language follow from the change in paradigms. On the biomedical model one tracks the progression of the disease by noting increasing levels of *functional impairment*. The degree of functional impairment might be measured and documented by appropriate healthcare professionals, perhaps by the patient's performance on one of the quality-of-life instruments previously noted. Most likely the progress would be noted in terms of the patient's ability to perform daily functions or to demonstrate independence. However, if one approaches the patient from the perspective of illness, then what becomes important is the patient's *subjective disablement*. "While measures of impairment may indicate deterioration, the individual's perceived disability may remain stable or improve." (Lyman, 1998, p. 51). From the perspective of subjective disablement, the limits and barriers may stem more from the social and physical environment than from the progression of the disease. For individuals experiencing dementia, chief among the social sources of disability is ineffective treatment by well-intentioned carers who too quickly deny them their status as persons through applying the labels "child-like" or "vegetable" and subverting their independence through what Lyman calls, quoting Luborsky (1994), "the tyranny of small decisions" (p. 51). Further, the biomedical model focuses on *decision making*, relying heavily on judgments of competence; the sociomedical approach is more concerned with *empowerment*, encouraging "persons with dementia to live life as fully as possible on their own terms" (Lyman, 1998, p. 52).

Finally, the biomedical tradition emphasizes that parts of the self are lost when a particular part of the person is lost. Lyman urges that we cease focusing on *loss-of-self* and address instead the importance of *creating meaning* in the lives of Alzheimer's patients. As the stories in the sections that follow illustrate, the creation of meaning is a daily phenomenon for individuals with dementia. In interpretive phenomenology humans are viewed as "meaning makers" through and through. Locating the metaphysical source of identity and selfhood is not important phenomenologically. What is important is the ongoing effort to create meaning in a world of discontinuity. As the impairment increases, Alzheimer's patients may not be able to find their identity internally; yet, despite the impairment, the meaning they continue to create staves off their disability. In the long run, it may be necessary to ground meaning in the narrative of their lives, though their grasp of that narrative may become more and more tenuous for them. We conclude this section of our chapter with a consideration of the importance of narrative.

When the biomedical model of health predominates, therapeutic interventions become generalized. If the disease is caused by a physiological condition, then similar diseases will receive similar therapies. Care is individuated only to the extent that there are discernible physiological differences that justify corresponding differences in dosage. In the absence of a personal relationship between the patient and the healthcare worker, there is no basis for personalized care. Rich (1996) argues that a values history based on the narrative of a patient's life can be the basis of personalized care for individuals in long-term care facilities. Individuals suffering from dementia live a life that becomes increasingly fragmented. As the dementia worsens, the individual loses the ability to provide the context within which events, thoughts, and actions receive meaning. But the loss of memory, according to Rich, does not mean loss of identity. He asserts:

Memories alone are not constitutive of continuing consciousness or personal identity. What is left out of this view [of personal identity] is the whole realm of mental states and dispositions which form a seamless web in the life of a single person when viewed from a narrative perspective. In this realm we find thoughts, ideas, beliefs, emotions, values, and aspirations. It is from these that a person derives her [sic] traits of character and personality that make her a unique individual who endures through time and changing circumstances. (p. 77)

Rich (1996) locates personal identity in the "enduring virtues (and vices), values, priorities, and predilections which shape one's character and personality" (p. 78). It is just this dimension of ourselves that allows each of us to respond uniquely to the challenges of disease and to be aware of our illnesses and disabilities. He recommends that a values history become as much a part of a patient's record as a medical history for it "ascertains the primary values that have governed a patient's life." (p. 78). The values history helps to provide meaning and context to a patient's narratives and provides a basis for continuing to make decisions in keeping with those values even when the individual can no longer provide continuity, through articulated memory, to the ongoing biography.

Part 2. Power, Oppression, and Quality of Life of Persons With Dementia

Perceptions of quality of life provide an underpinning for many interventions in long-term care. In caring for patients with chronic degenerative diseases, health professionals may see prolonging of life and use of expensive resources as futile if the quality of life of these patients is deemed to be poor. A key question is, "Given this quality of life, what ought we to do?" Thus, it is vital that health professionals begin to question traditional understandings of quality of life and to explore multiple perspectives on this phenomenon—particularly the perspectives of patients and families living with a chronic degenerative disease.

Part 1 of this chapter introduced concepts related to quality of life that challenge our traditional assumptions about this phenomenon. The biomedicalization of aging, and specifically of chronic diseases such as Alzheimer's Disease, have focused health professionals' clinical gaze on *disease,* rather than the *illness* experience (Brody, 1987; Hahn, 1995). With this model, aging is viewed as itself a pathology, with an inevitable process of decline, impairment, degeneration, and death. The reduction of illness to disease leads healthcare professionals to conclude that they are in the best position to make meaningful judgments about interventions and provides them the legitimate power to act as decision makers for patients.

As discussed in part 1, Moody (1992) helps us see the usefulness of an alternative model for understanding quality of life. This model adopts a hermeneutic approach to focus on the context and meaning embedded in an individual's experience with illness. Meanings are always situated in historical contexts. Lyman (1998) uses a similar approach in discussing how older people may negotiate their social relationships and individual identities to incorporate the changes associated with chronic illness. She emphasizes that we need to pay attention to the viewpoints of those who have lived with the extremes of impairment, loss, and dependency.

This section of the chapter extends our discussion to consider how a historical context, viewed as life narratives, can help us to understand the illness experience of persons with Alzheimer's Disease. Excerpts from an ongoing phenomenological study of ethical concerns of persons with Alzheimer's Disease, as well as their family members and professional carers, are interpreted within the framework of the power of the healthcare system and the power of the healthcare provider in relation to these individuals' own life narratives.

Life Narratives as Interpretation in the Context of Illness

We believe that restrictive interpretations of quality of life may lead to oppression and violence through failure by health professionals to take into account the patient's narrative of his or her life. Coles (1989) says that "the people who come to see us bring us their stories. . . . They hope they tell them well enough so that we understand the truth of their lives" (p. 7). Listening to narratives of persons with dementia within the context of their past, values, and relationships is critical to extending our interpretations of quality of life. Narratives are increasingly being seen as an approach to understanding the unique perspective of a patient living with an illness, not merely a disease (Sacks, 1985).

Coles (1989), a prominent child psychiatrist, notes that as health professionals, we are trained to get to the heart of "the problem" quickly in dialogues with patients—to reduce the information obtained from patients to a coherent, concise note that can be entered in their health records. We expect structured presentations and sometimes become impatient if these do not materialize as we anticipated. Coles describes how his mentor helped him to move away from taking "case histories" of patients. Only then, Coles notes, did he begin to understand the illness experiences of his patients.

Life narratives are formed through the process of blending an individual's life-long thoughts, emotions, spiritual explorations, and actions. These narratives evolve through one's life, through the process of living. Too often, we fragment these narratives into disjointed segments, such as childhood, adulthood, and old age (Rich, 1996). In this way, the distinctiveness of each segment, rather than the unity of the narrative, holds our gaze. Some Alzheimer's patients may be seen as moving backward into time, back to the dependency of childhood. Within this perspective, the individual with increasing severity of dementia and decreasing mental and physical function may be seen by those unaware of an individual's narrative history as devoid of any meaningful quality of life.

Yet, there is a persisting self that has traversed this passage through distinct stages of life (Rich, 1996). This self is not a new identity. Instead, it is a new blending of previous narratives, forming a new configuration that can be viewed from different perspectives. As humans, we are always already becoming our possibilities. We need to acknowledge that one possibility for us as humans may be Alzheimer's Disease. Sorting through the narratives of our lives is analogous to looking through a kaleidoscope, where as we turn the focusing ring, the perceived images change in texture and appearance. The pieces of colored glass themselves do not change—only the way they merge to form an image. But unlike the kaleidoscope that constructs many beautiful images, the resultant images with Alzheimer's Disease and other dementias are often seen as ugly and distasteful, rather than one of the possibilities of living a life.

The blending of life narratives in a person living with Alzheimer's Disease can be viewed, collectively, as a coming to be of memories. A poem by Heidegger (1971, p. 10) engages us in thinking about how memories are integrated into our life narratives:

The oldest of the old follows behind
    us in our thinking and yet it
    comes to meet us.
That is why thinking holds to the
    coming of what has been, and
    is remembrance.

A poignant example of how memories are integrated into life narratives is presented by the British literary critic John Bayley (1999) in his memoir about his wife, Iris Murdoch, a prominent novelist who became progressively impaired with Alzheimer's Disease. The book weaves together the reflections of a loving and articulate husband who never felt alone, even when his wife failed to recognize him, because of his memories of the narratives they had shared together. Bayley contrasts his personal reflections with the perceptions of society as he describes two experiences, 30 years apart, when he and Iris shared a swim in a river:

With the ardour of comparative youth, we wormed our way through the rank grass and sedge until we almost fell into it. Crouching in the shelter of the reeds, we tore our clothes off and slipped in like water rats. . . . A moment after we had crawled out and were drying ourselves on Iris's half-slip a big pleasure boat chugged past within a few feet of the bank. The steersman, wearing a white cap, gazed intently ahead. (p. 4)

Bayley then describes a second swim, 30 years later:

Our own little nook was seldom occupied, and it was empty today, as usual. Once, we would have got our clothes off as soon as possible and slid silently into the water, as we had done on that first occasion. Now I had quite a struggle getting Iris's clothes off: I had managed to put her bathing suit on at home, before we started. . . . [Now] she protested, gently though vigorously, as I tugged off the outer layers. In her shabby old one-piece swimsuit . . . she was an awkward and anxious figure, her socks trailing around her ankles. She was obstinate about not taking these off, and I gave up the struggle. A pleasure barge chugged slowly past, an elegant girl in a bikini sunning herself on the deck, a young man in white shorts at the steering wheel. Both turned to look at us with a slight air of incredulity. I should not have been surprised if they had burst into guffaws of ill-mannered laughter, for we must have presented a comic spectacle—an elderly man struggling to remove the garments from an old lady, still with white skin and incongruously fair hair. (pp. 36–37)

Rich (1996) emphasizes the distinction between "being alive" and "having a life." Persons in a persistent vegetative state are alive in a biological sense because they do not yet meet the prescribed criteria for death. Having a life, however, is a very different concept. Having a life means living a life that can be understood and appreciated *biographically*. Dementia does not necessarily mean the end to a biographical life. All humans *are* a history, which is reflected in life narratives. This is neither lost nor denied by the presence of Alzheimer's Disease. Even in dementia, a biographical life can be created and recreated through life narratives. Bayley helps us to glimpse this biographical essence of a life in his description of how he and Iris created a rich life together, even after she was severely impaired with Alzheimer's Disease. Bayley also presents a poignant contrast between his own perceptions of aging and of caring for a beloved wife with Alzheimer's and the way that society sees these conditions of life.

Ethical Issues in the Care of Persons With Alzheimer's Disease

Excerpts from an ongoing phenomenological study of ethical issues related to the care of persons with Alzheimer's Disease are used here to reflect the potential for violence when perspectives of quality of life described by Alzheimer's patients and their families are dismissed (Sorrell, 2000). The study gathered perspectives of persons with Alzheimer's Disease, as well as their family members and professional carers. The *Fairhill Guidelines on Ethics and the Care of People With Alzheimer's Disease* (Post & Whitehouse, 1995) provided a framework for the study. These guidelines were the culmination of discussions among a diverse group of professionals, including nurses, physicians, lawyers, ethicists, and administrators, who gathered monthly from October 1993 through June 1994 to listen to stories of family carers and individuals with mild dementia of the Alzheimer's type. The overall purpose of these sessions was to address ethical concerns related to dementia care. These *Fairhill Guidelines* provide a starting point for health professionals to reconsider assumptions related to the quality of life of persons with dementia. Health professionals must recognize that any "measurement" of quality of life includes a subjectivity that no outward observer can assess. One family carer in the *Fairhill Guidelines* discussions believed that people often assess the quality of life of an Alzheimer's person more negatively than justified because of the high regard for cognitive skills and productivity in our society (Post & Whitehouse). She noted that her severely demented father could play a game of cards long after he forgot who she was and found moments of real joy in this activity. She warns: "We intellectuals are not a jury of dad's peers" (Post & Whitehouse, p. 1427).

For the Sorrell (2000) study, ethical issues embedded in the *Fairhill Guidelines* discussions were used to design an unstructured interview tool that focused on five areas: (a) truthtelling; (b) autonomy; (c) behavior control; (d) death and dying; and (e) quality of life. A snowball method of sampling was used to identify participants for interviews in the study. Criteria included: (a) participants had experienced Alzheimer's Disease as a patient, family member, or professional carer, and (b) participants could discuss their perspectives in English. Data presented here are drawn from 16 interviews: 4 of these interviews were with persons with an early diagnosis of Alzheimer's Disease, and 10 interviews were with family members. Two additional interviews were carried out with a nurse and physician who specialize in the care of persons with Alzheimer's Disease.

All participants in the study were asked to describe critical incidents that stood out in their minds about ethical issues they had experienced in day-to-day living with Alzheimer's Disease. Prompts were used during the interviews to identify ethical concerns related to the five categories from the *Fairhill Guidelines* listed previously. All interviews were audiotaped and transcribed verbatim. Narrative summaries were written of interviews. Excerpts presented here are focused around: (a) the power of the healthcare system; (b) the power of the healthcare provider; and (c) life narratives of persons with Alzheimer's Disease.

The Power of the Healthcare System

Too often, healthcare professionals, using a standard of functional competence and lacking a sense of the patient's life narrative, may determine that a patient has a poor quality of life. Human thought and action are made intelligible by placing them within the context of the life of an individual. When health professionals perceive that a patient's quality of life has hopelessly deteriorated, they may do violence by fragmenting the unity of this person's life into disjointed segments. Thus, health professionals have a moral obligation to rethink the assumptions that underlie their definitions of quality of life. Considering patients only in the immediate present cuts them off from their past, values, and relationships—from those very things that form their life narrative.

One family carer interviewed in the study, Pamela, talked about the sense of injustice that she felt her father-in-law experienced when he suffered a stroke at home. He had been cared for by his family physician over the 8 years of progression of his Alzheimer's Disease. Now, at 90, he was frail but had been living in his home on an island with assistance of two aides who came to his home twice a day to help with medication administration and other chores. Pamela, a nurse, recognized the symptoms of previous small strokes and the transient paralysis of her father-in-law's left extremities. At the time of the 2000 Republican Convention, he suffered a more severe stroke that caused him to fall and lose consciousness. Pamela attempted to persuade the physician to admit her father-in-law to the hospital for tests, but the physician refused. Instead, he advised placement in a nursing home. Pamela describes her frustrations:

It made me so angry, for President Ford had a stroke on almost the same day, and he was hospitalized. In fact, he's still there, days later. But, of course, President Ford is an important person with intact cognitive abilities. My father-in-law is not an important person to society; he's old and frail and demented. Yet, if he had been hospitalized, he could have been tested to see if there were treatments that could improve his quality of life related to these strokes in his last days. Also, hospital admission would have meant that his first 90 days in the nursing home would have been covered. But no one thought he was important enough. (Sorrell, 2000)

As noted in part 1 of this chapter, the attraction to the use of QALYs in healthcare economics reflects the assumption that introducing scientific measures and procedures can determine the right course of action in a more objective manner. QALYs are intended to reflect the extent to which certain healthcare interventions cost-effectively produce benefits greater than the suffering that may accompany them. In a managed-care environment, resources are distributed to provide the most cost-effective use. If persons with dementia are seen as of little value, healthcare providers may determine that expensive resources should not be "wasted" on them.

Looking at quality of life through the preconceptions and power of the healthcare system, rather than the individual patient's or family's perspective, may undermine decision making related to quality of life. For example, Pamela's father-in-law, although frail, was in fairly good physical health when he experienced his stroke. Also, the paralysis from the stroke was transient, leaving him with no serious physical deficits. Pamela was asking only for a reasonable evaluation of her father-in-law's condition to identify potential areas focused around his stroke that could be treated. This certainly would have been the accepted practice for a younger and/or cognitively aware person.

At present, the power of the healthcare system resides in the healthcare providers as decision makers, not in the patients and families. Especially in the present context of scarce resources, healthcare providers must learn to practice medical decision making as a dialogue between themselves, patients, and families—a conversation that leaves open possibilities. We cannot know what *should* be done unless we question our assumptions about quality of life and learn to listen to the life narratives of patients and families.

Even the language we use provides clues to the power inherent in the healthcare system. We talk of "placing" someone in a nursing home, as if we are dealing with an object or "nonperson." Almost all of the carers in the research study talked of how wrenching the decision was to have to consider placement of their loved one in a nursing home. It is ironic that our society tends to frown on family members' decisions to place a loved one in a nursing home yet provides minimal help in securing alternative approaches. Literature addressing reasons for placement in a nursing home suggests that there are multiple influences besides physical or mental impairment that determine whether a person is admitted to a nursing home. Some of these determining factors are regional, ethnic, and gender variations and conditions and problems of the carer support system (Congdon & Magilvy, 1998; Cox, 1986; Ferrucci, Guralnik, Pahor, Corti, & Havlik, 1997). When listening to narratives of illness, it becomes apparent that health professionals' perspectives on quality of life may be important determinants for nursing home placement.

Paul, the son of the 90-year-old man with Alzheimer's described previously, is a doctorally prepared social worker and health policy analyst. He described how he had to push the system as hard as he could, "and then still a bit more," to obtain what he believed that his father needed to maintain the best quality of life. Paul talked about how over 8 years he had worked to solve one problem after another so that his father could maintain his independence in his own home. He notes:

I had this idea, I guess it was inherited from my mother and grandmother, that the best way to die was to die in one's own bed. To me, it was the ideal I held for my father. I don't know, maybe it's an Irish thing, but it was important to me. So I did everything I could possibly think of to keep him living independently in his home. Even up until now, I think he had a good quality life. His only loss of quality in his life was his recognition that his abilities to live alone were gradually disappearing. It wasn't his quality of life that was the problem: it was securing the resources from the healthcare system so that he could maintain that quality of life as long as possible. I'm well educated and I know how to push the buttons, and I do. One day, after waiting on the phone forever listening to Muzak, trying to get approval from the HMO for my father's cataract surgery, I got angry and called the President of the HMO. I got approval. But what do less educated people without any knowledge of the health system do? They're left to try to figure out whether to push 1, 2, 10 or whatever to try to get service—and then they may not even be able to understand English. (Sorrell, 2000)

The interviewer was amazed to realize that this 90-year-old man with progressive and severe dementia had been able to live independently in his home, on an island, for over 8 years. Most persons in similar circumstances probably would have been placed in a nursing home much earlier. This son, however, was someone who valued problem solving and was expert at it. Even in the absence of the voice of the father, he believed that he understood the narrative identity of his father and how it defined the quality of life for him. Probably, if Paul's father had been asked, years earlier, to complete one of the quality-of-life questionnaires described by Gill and Feinstein (1994), he would have scored poorly. After all, the functional capacities measured by these tools were severely limited. Yet, with creative and aggressive acquisition of health resources by his son, he was able to maintain a quality of life valued by him and his son.

A healthcare system that ignores the life narratives of patients and families may do violence to their own perspectives of quality of life, leading to decisions by healthcare providers that fail to consider the context of the patient's illness experience. Thus, healthcare providers need to learn to attend to these life narratives in their interpretations of quality of life.

The Power of the Healthcare Provider

As health professionals, it is tempting to bemoan our lack of power. After all, it is managed care that controls so much of access and use of healthcare resources. Yet, we are able to secure the best resources for "high tech," acute care for patients. We are trained to use technology to help patients improve, to change. Yet, it is important to guard against being claimed by technology. What happens if we cannot improve a patient's condition? Does this mean the patient has less value?

In a society that places a high value on memory, intellectual abilities, and economic productivity, it is vital that health professionals reflect on how these values affect individuals with dementia. Cultural undercurrents tend to diminish the moral significance of people with dementia. Because we value rationality and productivity, we may see the life of a person with dementia as lacking worth. Too often, the loss of cognition that occurs in dementia is equated with hopelessness and uselessness. This perception leads to what Post (1995) refers to as "exclusionary ethics": too great a value placed on rationality and memory excludes individuals with dementia from the sphere of human dignity and respect and leaves them socially marginalized.

Alzheimer's patients may not improve. Sophisticated technology is not likely to make an impact on these persons as their cognitive abilities continue to degenerate. The stunning advances in medical technology in such areas as transplants, infertility, and even, increasingly, AIDS seem to have bypassed those with Alzheimer's Disease. Too often the course is a slowly progressive dementia that leaves the patient cognitively incapacitated and the carers and families financially, physically, and emotionally depleted. Nurses, physicians, and other health professionals must help carers understand how to solve problems that may seem insurmountable. This type of power is grounded in listening and human connections, not technology.

Nancy, a nurse who works with persons with Alzheimer's in a day-care center, put it this way:

Lots of people feel that this person is misbehaving on purpose, that they could control it, they could change if they tried. Families think that way, if they just would, you know, just sit there for five minutes. Well, they can't sit there for five minutes. I mean, the disease is changing the person. It's not the person not wanting to do what you're asking, they just can't do it anymore. (Sorrell, 2000)

Although listening to others is the hallmark of an anthropological perspective and practice, the inevitable cultural gap between healthcare professionals and patients makes this difficult (Hahn, 1995). Understanding the experience of living with dementia requires an intimate type of relationship between health professional, patient, and family that is unusual in today's healthcare system. In our fast-paced and technologically sophisticated society, we may not want to take time to listen, a condition that Fiumara (1990) refers to as "benumbment" (p. 84). In the midst of the constant noise of our modern world, we need to create sufficient silence to hear ourselves and others. As noted in part 1 of this chapter, in an earlier, less complex time the relationship of the physician to the patient was usually based on long experience and intimate knowledge of both the patient and family. With a close and continuing relationship based on knowledge and trust, health professionals are in a good position to listen and to advocate for their patients. But as noted by Paul, the social worker who discussed his father's care, this is a rare occurrence today:

Who knows their patients today? When I was in practice, I always made sure that when I made a referral, it was received at the other end. In those days, we didn't just assume it would happen. Today my students in social work don't see the need for that. Physicians, too, used to know how to advocate for their patients. With the fragmented nature of managed care today, this seems almost impossible. (Sorrell, 2000)

The healthcare provider does have power—the power of guiding decision making within a managed care environment that includes attention not only to QALYs but also to the need to implement listening practices in healthcare as one way to overcome oppression. Health professionals need to listen to the narratives of patients and families so that they can effectively advocate for them. John, who has cared for his mother with Alzheimer's Disease, put it this way:

I think we all have an individual responsibility, and society has a responsibility, to care for those who can't care for themselves. And whether that's the beginning of life or the end of life, wherever life is vulnerable, we've got to care for it in a loving way. . . . From an ethics point of view, we want to make sure, or I want to be part of a society that values vulnerable life. And we're talking about people that are terribly vulnerable but who are all loved. And that's the bottom line here I think. (Sorrell, 2000)

Life Narratives of Persons with Alzheimer's Disease

One key to understanding ethical care for persons with dementia is appreciating noncognitive aspects of human well-being. Health professionals must learn how to call forth storytelling—to make innovative space to listen attentively to patients and carers, acknowledging the context of the situation and the necessity to ground interpretations of quality of life in concrete experience. This approach to ethics, rather than relying on traditional principles, encourages dialogue with those with dementia and their carers to define what aspects of the illness are morally important. Through listening to narratives of lived experiences, we can reshape our image of people with dementia so that ethical analysis is transformed. Through a focus on interpretation of the experience of dementia, we can help to establish an ethics of respect for the individual experience, spiritual meanings, and dignity of those affected.

Nancy provides her impression of quality of life in dementia, based on years of experience of working as a nurse in a respite center for persons with Alzheimer's Disease:

I think the gray area for me, is what is end-of-life for a person with dementia? We have people here who are in the very late stages of Alzheimer's Disease, and maybe from an objective standpoint, you could say, "Well, what is their quality of life? Somebody has to feed this person, somebody has to transfer this person from the chair to the commode, somebody has to get this person dressed in the morning. What quality of life are you talking about?" And yet, when you see, you know the music gets turned on, and you see the person enjoying the music and holding a grandchild or . . . holding a dog and petting it, things like that, those experiences are the same kinds of things that give us joy. (Sorrell, 2000)

Patients in nursing homes deeply miss the availability of meaningful activities, causing them to lose a sense of purpose and adopt a negative self-image (Post, 1995). Too often, long-term care settings cut off the self from the narrative unity of the life that came before. An ethical approach in long-term care must honor patients' life narratives. The biographical life they continue, in spite of dementia, is something about which they care deeply. Bayley (1999) noted this: "I've come to realize, among Alzheimer's partners [that] one needs very much to feel that the unique individuality of one's spouse has not been lost in the common symptoms of a clinical condition" (p. 49).

Family carers of Alzheimer patients sometimes describe quality of life as "quality of lives," emphasizing the personal identity of an individual formed within the context of connections with loved ones (Post & Whitehouse, 1995). When a life is viewed through a narrative perspective, the connections of various stages in the life process can be seen to contribute to the unity of the life and to the individual's personal identity. Healthcare professionals need to widen the lens through which they view quality of life and identify ways to understand the life narratives of patients and their families.

Carers interviewed in the study talked of the meanings embedded in their caregiving experiences. Kitwood pointed out a connection between caregiving and its aesthetic reflection on our humanity. He stated that to respond "appropriately to a person's needs . . . is to create something that is beautiful" (Ferenz, 2000, p. 69). It appears that carers may spend their lives reliving memories of their caregiving. Heidegger describes memory as not merely "thinking back to something thought," but also "the gathering of recollection" (Heidegger, 1977, p. 376). He notes that memory "safely keeps and keeps concealed within it that to which at any given time thought must first be given in everything that essentially unfolds, appealing to us as what has being and has been in being" (p. 376). The memories of carers in the study often poured forth with tears. Many said that they had not talked to anyone of these reflections; they had kept them safely concealed from others. Some expressed regret that, in spite of all their efforts, they had not been able to do enough for their loved one. Health professionals must find a way to help families safely articulate these memories of caregiving experiences. Interpretive phenomenology can help to point out the importance of such life narratives. Healthcare providers need to learn to attend to them.

Bill, a participant in the study who has cared for his wife with Alzheimer's for many years, described the agonizing decisions he deals with on a daily basis and how difficult it is to balance these with his devotion to his wife:

One of the problems that arises out of all this is that she recognizes how tough it is on me, more than she recognizes how tough it is on her. And two or three times a week, she'll come to me and say, "We've got to talk about me going into some kind of a care facility," and then we have, "No, we can't do that, I can't live without you." And these kinds of things hurt me emotionally. And it hurts her emotionally. But it is always overhanging us there, and we don't know when, as I've told her, I don't know when that time will come, but when it comes, I'll know it. But until then, we're going to be together. And I'm your caregiver. (Sorrell, 2000)

Bill's story reveals caring practices that are often embedded in narratives of caregiving, such as awaiting, accompanying, and bearing witness. Post (1995) suggests that the moral role of the family is to create a framework of value and a sphere of care that bears witness to the value and worth of a loved one with dementia (p. 42). The long progression over time of a disease such as Alzheimer's requires an "awaiting" by the carers, who bear witness to the creative possibilities inherent in caregiving. Bill's story portrays the solicitude of caregiving as he describes how he accompanies his wife in her journey through dementia, awaiting "that time" that he knows will come. Bill, like many carers, was able to reconstitute meanings that accompany his awaiting. Too often, however, these meanings lie invisible and fallow within the caregiving experience. The French philosopher Gabriel Marcel wrote of care as "the mystery of presence" (Post, 1995, p. 8). In the biomedical model, health professionals are often intent on "doing to," rather than "being with." Health professionals need to learn what type of meaningful care they can provide for families in the awaiting time. How can they bear witness to the creative possibilities that these families bring to their caregiving? New models must be implemented in healthcare that create a space for storytelling and conversation, so that the practices of solicitude embedded in caregiving narratives can be called forth.

Sacks (1985) has noted that only when we see persons in their own worlds can we appreciate the depths of their experiences. Health professionals usually encounter Alzheimer patients in an environment very different from the patients' own worlds, making it imperative to make efforts to understand their everyday experiences in their own worlds. Research suggests that, even in advanced dementia, persons are capable of thoughtful, protective, emotional, sensitive, and empathetic interactions with others (Russell, 1996). Listening to narratives of patients and their carers can help us to understand others' perspectives of quality of life and to identify ways to foster humanistic interventions appropriate to a specific context of care.

Mac, another study participant, describes the satisfying relationship he has maintained with his wife with Alzheimer's even after she entered a nursing home. It is clear that he has thought carefully about her quality of life. He keeps open a future of possibilities, yet does not sentimentalize her illness:

It pleases me to go visit her. . . . In fact, I think frequently about my visits, and people say it must be awfully hard on you to go visit. It's not. It's enjoyable to go visit with her, even though there's very little between us. But I don't want to prolong the situation artificially. When her time comes, I want it to come naturally. (Sorrell, 2000)

When a life is viewed through narratives, the stages of life become connected with these narratives, effecting a unity of the life and contributing to the individual's personal identity, as well as to the shared identity of patient with family carers. The extension of perspectives of quality of life in dementia to incorporate quality of lives emphasizes the humanhood of an individual formed within the context of connections with loved ones in one's life.

John describes the rather surprising possibilities he has uncovered in the relationship that has evolved over the years of caring for his mother with Alzheimer's:

I love her intensely, and her conversation's playful, and when I go visit her now, my only intent is to enjoy her, and not try to get her to do something. And it's a relationship I've never had with my mother, and I wouldn't trade that for anything, anything, no matter what happens. (Sorrell, 2000)

Excerpts from participants in the research on ethics in the care of persons with Alzheimer's Disease reveal the need for an alternative model in healthcare that attends to the context and meaning embedded in human experience. Failure to understand a person's biographical life can lead to restricted interpretations of quality of life, which in turn can lead to oppression and violence. Health professionals need to develop caring practices that provide creative space for storytelling, conversation, and listening to bring forth the life narratives that constitute their persons.

Part 3. Personhood, Spirituality, and Quality of Life of Persons With Dementia

In this part of the chapter, we specifically argue that attention to a spiritual dimension with its concern for meaning and integration (Hiatt, 1995) can enhance the lives of persons with dementia and their families. In this regard, the questions we raise are these: Should persons with severe dementia, because of their dementia, be viewed as less than human? or as lacking spirituality? Our position is that they should not be viewed in these ways. Other scholars (Fletcher, 1972, 1974; Shelp, 1986; Veatch, 1993) disagree and would argue that persons with severe dementia are incapable of fulfilling the criteria for personhood or for maintaining spirituality. Such a position, we believe, diminishes a person's moral status, thus, potentially inflicting violence and harm. We now examine both sides of the preceding questions as they relate to violence, quality of life, and spirituality.

The Case Against Personhood

The case against personhood, simply put, is that if an individual lacks one or more of the essential qualities of personhood, for example, capacity for rational thought and/or cognitive functioning, for meaning-making, and for recognition of others, then the individual is not or is no longer a person. The implications of denying personhood can be seen in the following argument: (a) If the cognitive, meaning-making, and recognition parts of a person are lacking, that constitutes a sufficient reason to deny personhood; (b) if individuals are not persons, they lack moral status; (c) lack of moral status justifies treating an individual differently, in particular, denying them certain fundamental rights and privileges (e.g., right to life). In addition, individuals who are denied the moral status of persons are unlikely to be viewed as experiencing a spiritual dimension.

Without realizing it, healthcare professionals and families of persons with dementia too often use labels that devalue individuals with dementia. How often have you heard the following labels referring to an individual with dementia? "Loss of self," "loss of prior self," "a living death," "a shell of one's former self," "just like kids again," "like a vegetable now," "AD victim," or "we can just keep the person comfortable" (Holstein, 1998; Lyman, 1998; McCurdy, 1998). In addition to labeling, Kitwood (1998) focuses on actual interpersonal practices of healthcare providers that oppress and do violence to the personhood and narrative identities of individuals with dementia. These interpersonal practices include deception, disempowerment, infantilization, intimidation, stigmatization, outpacing, invalidation, banishment, objectification, ignoring, imposition, withholding, accusation, disruption, mockery, and disparagement.

The preceding labels or interpersonal practices either decontextualize persons with dementia from the predementia narratives of their lives or demean them in their current state. Regardless, labels or practices such as these oppress persons with dementia by creating an unequal power balance and by dehumanizing them. Furthermore, carers must understand that interpersonal relationships are indeed practices and not intentions. What matters is not what I intend to do or say but what I in fact do and say. As a result, those who use these expressions or engage in these interactions, often unthinkingly, cause harm to persons with dementia in the name of quality of life; "They do not yet appreciate the redeeming words, 'I am' " (Post, 1995, p. 18).

The following two stories show how apparently reasonable nursing care based on the biomedical model failed as a result of decontextualizing persons with dementia and, as a result, led to their oppression.

ETHEL

Ethel had been in an assisted-living apartment for some time, but when her dependency became too great for her to continue there, a place was found for her in residential care. She had a very comfortable room, with toilet and bathroom facilities *en suite*. Ethel settled in well, and with her pleasant, sociable personality soon became a popular figure with her fellow residents. A problem, however, was occurring in her room: Each night Ethel urinated on the carpet. When the night staff tried to get her to go to the toilet before she went to bed she refused, sometimes angrily. Each morning the carpet was wet, and soon the room began to smell of urine. Ethel's son Peter, who visited regularly, was very upset at what he found, and complained to the manager of the home. So the efforts to rectify Ethel's toiletting behavior were intensified. The staff reminded Ethel repeatedly about the *en suite* facilities, and left the light on [*sic*] in the toilet at night. None of these measures, however, were successful. Some of the staff began to feel deeply resentful. They criticized Ethel for being lazy, and this lowered her morale. The only feasible solution seemed to be to put Ethel into incontinence pads. (Kitwood, 1998, p. 25)

MAY AND DOROTHY

May and her sister Dorothy had been admitted into residential care together. May was extremely dependent and demanding, and Dorothy carried the main burden. After Dorothy died this pattern of behavior intensified; also May tended to be extremely rude to staff members, often making abusive remarks such as "You bitch." She also spent long periods shouting out "Help me, help me," in very public places such as the foyer or the lounge. At first some of the staff tried to respond kindly to May and to discover what she was really asking for; May, however, seemed unable to explain. Others were less sensitive, and made comments such as "If you don't want anything, why do you continually ask for help?" May's behavior was generally perceived as being symptomatic of her dementia, without any attempt at a deeper understanding. Various attempts were made to "modify her behavior," particularly by ignoring her when she was shouting—but to no avail. May came to be disliked by almost everyone. (Kitwood, 1998, p. 26)

The preceding two stories demonstrate violation of the ethical principle of respect for persons. In Ethel's story, the staff assumed that she was purposely being lazy by not using her bathroom facilities *en suite* and urinating on the carpet instead. The staff did all they perceived they could do to rectify the problem but without success; some staff then began to deeply resent Ethel. These staff were, initially, unable to "see" her toileting problems through a lens that provided a perspective on her previous experiences.

In May's story, violation of the ethical principle of respect for persons became a problem because the staff members, who at first responded kindly to May, were unable to alter her crying-out behavior. The staff members were satisfied to view it as symptomatic of her dementia. They, too, were unable to see her crying-out behavior through a new lens or to see its connection to her narrative identity.

This new phenomenological lens has been introduced previously (Lyman, 1998) and is reviewed here. In both Ethel's and in May's stories, the staff initially operated within the biomedical model as discussed in part 1 of our chapter. There we noted the significance of emphasizing disease in contrast to illness, functional impairment in contrast to disablement, decision making in contrast to empowerment, and loss of self in contrast to creation of meaning. The staff viewed each situation from their own perspectives rather than that of Ethel and May. Unaware of Ethel's and May's life narratives, the staff lacked criteria for interpreting the meaning of their actions.

The staff's point of view is understandable as this is the way many were taught to conceptualize healthcare within the medical model. Most likely, it would not enter the staff member's minds that their actions violated the ethical principle of respect for persons and, in doing so, diminished the moral status of Ethel and of May. Such diminishing devalues patients and increases the potential for oppression and violence. As a result, persons with dementia suffer loss of quality of life because their self-identity has been eroded.

The Case for Personhood

The case for personhood, simply put, is that an individual with dementia should not be viewed as fragmented or reduced to component parts but rather is to be viewed as a whole person. This definition or similar ones have considerable support in the current literature (e.g., Holstein, 1998; Kapp, 1998; Kitwood, 1997, 1998; Lyman, 1998; McCurdy, 1998; Nelson, 1998; Post, 1995, 1998; Sabat, 1998). As noted previously, Lyman offers a phenomenological perspective that is based on the lived experience and life narrative of a person with dementia. Thus, quality of life takes on a new meaning because it is "patient" focused and not "other" focused, and because the subjectivity of the experience is deemed as an acceptable criterion for defining quality of life.

We now complete the stories of Ethel and of May by discussing interventions that respected their personhood. The interventions enhanced the quality of Ethel's and May's lives after the staff viewed each situation through the patient's lens.

ETHEL—THE REST OF THE STORY

One staff member, however, made a crucial observation. This was that Ethel always urinated in the same place, near the head of the bed. He asked Peter to tell him exactly what the arrangements had been in Ethel's former apartment. Peter said that Ethel had had a commode, close by her bed. A commode was provided for Ethel in her new room, and immediately all was well; Ethel used it every night. The "toiletting problems" disappeared. The goodwill of staff toward Ethel returned, and with that her social confidence was restored. (Kitwood, 1998, pp. 25–26)

MAY—THE REST OF THE STORY

A small research team was spending time in the home, and they put forward a new hypothesis. Perhaps May's cry of "Help me, help me," really meant something like "Help me to find myself again." If so, she was pleading to be recognized and accepted as a real, unique person, and not asking for anything specific. So members of the research team started to give real attention to May; for example sitting with her, walking with her, and responding when she showed a need for physical contact. Slowly May began to show more signs of self-respect, taking greater interest in her appearance. She became more trusting, and less territorial about her chair. The repetitive shouting gradually subsided. . . . So May came to be acknowledged as a real human being, not a "dement," and some staff found that they genuinely liked her. The engaging and loving aspects of May's personality became apparent for all to see. (Kitwood, 1998, p. 26)

The rest of Ethel's and May's stories raise several questions. Regarding Ethel, why did the staff members react as they did, using some of the interpersonal practices (e.g., objectification, disparagement) decried by Kitwood (1998)? Why, initially, were the staff members unable to frame Ethel's toileting problems in a new way rather than to intensify the old routine way? Why did only one staff member make the observation that Ethel consistently urinated in the same spot? Why did some of the staff members disparage her by calling her lazy? Perhaps the night shift was understaffed and the amount of time they spent on her toileting behavior deprived other residents of the care that they needed. Perhaps the son's complaining to the manager of the home angered the staff. Whatever the reasons, until the problem was solved the care needed to maintain Ethel's psychological well-being was not provided. Initially the staff's practice failed because all but one staff member did not know what mattered to Ethel as a person and not as an object.

Regarding May, some similar questions also can be raised. Why did the staff's initial kindness toward May turn to disparagement and abandonment by some? Why were the staff members unable to see beyond her dementia, but the research team could? Did the research team exceed traditional research boundaries? Perhaps the staff members were so indoctrinated in the medical model of disease that they could not see beyond the symptoms of dementia. Perhaps the research team had more time to validate May's worth as a person.

In summary, then, the holistic and phenomenological position of personhood as illustrated in the preceding stories are based on the following argument developed by the authors: (a) The absence of the cognitive part of an individual should not necessarily deny personhood because a sense of self and meaning can be maintained through reconstitution; (b) if individuals are persons they possess moral status; and (c) moral status requires treating an individual as a person with fundamental rights and privileges. Further, individuals whose moral status is acknowledged are more likely to be viewed by staff as capable of experiencing a spiritual dimension.

Humanness, Spirituality, and Persons With Dementia

We have just reviewed arguments for and against personhood and examined how failing to acknowledge individuals as persons influences our view of their moral status and makes them vulnerable to oppressive and demeaning behavior. Historically, the philosophical analysis of personhood rests on a metaphysical claim about the presence or absence of certain critical qualities. From the perspective of interpretive phenomenology, we are more concerned with describing an experience than with establishing the reality of certain characteristics. In order to express the difference between the phenomenological and the metaphysical standpoints in this regard, we use the term *humanness* in the rest of this chapter to refer to the experiential dimension of individuals that makes it appropriate to recognize them as moral beings. We leave aside the metaphysical questions relating to the defining characteristics of persons in order to concentrate on the experience of a presence that is the focus of an individual's life narrative and that contributes to a sense of spirituality and depth of meaning.

We now examine two definitions of spirituality to consider how attention to spirituality enhances the quality of life of individuals with dementia. We believe it is important to explore notions of spirituality because of the recent emphasis on it in healthcare articles, books, and conferences, as well as our beliefs about its importance to enhancing quality of life for both healthcare providers and patients.

Definitions of spirituality. Spirituality wears a thousand faces while still remaining elusive. This point is documented in almost every book or article one reads on the topic. (For a review of 10 representative definitions of spirituality and its derivations, see the 1992 article by Emblen.) As McSherry and Draper (1998) note, "There is no single authoritative definition" (p. 683). We ask: Should there be one? We think not. Why? Because spirituality is an ineffable concept and, therefore, cannot be frozen in a definition. Like experience itself, it is always becoming and changing. What one may find sacred and worthy of revering is in a perpetual and nonlinear process of development. As such, spirituality is neither representational nor generalizable.

In a concept synthesis study in which Goldberg (1998) sought nurses' opinions and reviewed the literature surrounding spirituality, she found that the following phenomena emerged: "Meaning, presencing, empathy/compassion, giving hope, love, religion/transcendence, touch, and healing" (p. 836). At first, she saw these phenomena as falling into two categories: physical and emotional. Upon further reflection, she rejected the two categories as inappropriate for a holistic view of spirituality. She then collapsed the two categories into one, which she labeled *connection.*

Goldberg (1998) then elaborated on the concept of connection. She saw it as a relationship between two or more elements that could be physical or mental. She noted that the phenomenon of connection is in keeping with holistic nursing care and with the thinking of philosophers such as Buber. She also noted that the phenomenon of connection has a "goodness of fit" with nursing and related discipline theories. One limitation of Goldberg's study for our purposes is that her focus was on the nurse and not on persons with dementia and their families.

Therefore, her study raises some questions. Do the phenomena that emerged from Goldberg's (1998) study apply to the spirituality of persons with dementia and their families? What about the concept of connection? Because our experience of humanness includes a sense of self, meaning, and full moral status, we believe that Goldberg's phenomena apply to individuals with dementia and their families, with some adjustments made for the dementia. For example, regarding meaning, families of persons with dementia may be actively searching for it, whereas persons with dementia may be reconstituting meaning in accord with their illness and their life narratives. Regarding presencing, families of persons with dementia may be cognitively intact to persons with dementia, whereas persons with dementia may be emotionally present to them.

Waldfogel (1997) also sees connection as an element of spirituality, along with such concepts as *meaning and purpose in life* and *transcendence*. Regarding connection, Waldfogel believes that illness is a source of distress that can affect a person's relationship with others; the ill person often feels alienation. Waldfogel also believes that connection with other persons or with that which is sacred has the potential for healing.

Regarding meaning and purpose in life, Waldfogel (1997) sees spirituality as partly associated with coherence, and coherence, in turn, as providing personal meaning to one's life. This meaning brings integrity to a person's sense of self and events beyond self. The integrating function of spirituality, thus, helps buffer a person against change and uncertainty.

Regarding transcendence, Waldfogel (1997) sees it as "a profound and potentially transformative experience" (p. 965). Illness can be a transformative experience when the ill person is able to rise above a limiting condition and, as a result, feel part of something bigger than self, whether it be the cosmos or nature. Such an experience can be liberating if the person accepts the state of altered consciousness, which is often spiritual and beyond the "normal" status of being.

What implications do Waldfogel's (1997) elements of spirituality have for individuals with dementia and their families? Much of the literature speaks to connection with others as the singular most important factor in maintaining the humanness of persons with dementia. Connection can take many forms depending on the stage of the disease: affirmative talking with, advocating for, being with, praying with, caring about, caring for, playing with, respectful of, in-tuneness with, as well as a gentle touch and unconditional love. These actions obviously are not mutually exclusive, although all have the common goal of enhancing humanness and, thus, quality of life. However, if overall these actions are ignored, quality of life is not only diminished but also oppression or violence could occur.

You have already read examples of both the negative and positive aspects of connection in the stories of Ethel and May. Now let's "listen" to an affirming story about Leo and another May—both about 80 years of age; however, Leo has dementia and May, his sister and carer, does not:

[Leo's] first question was an unclear "Who am I?" May answers in a kind and jovial voice, "What do you mean, you know who you are. You're Leo. You were a boxer. You're my brother." Leo inquires, "Boxer? Was I?" "Yes, you were," responds May. "Where am I?" asks Leo. "In Cleveland, where you've been living for years," says May. "Mobile?" inquires Leo. "No, you were born in Mobile [Alabama], but now you're in Cleveland," states May. "Who am I?" repeats Leo. "What, you forgot again who you are? You're Leo, silly," May responds. "School, school. Who was my mama?" "Why you silly bones," answers May. "You know your mama was Leona, and she was my mama too, and you don't go to school." "Who am I?" Leo asks again. (Post, 1995, p. 8)

Although the cycle of questions and answers continues, Post (1995, p. 8) observed that Leo was not agitated about the repetitiveness of his questions because he was unaware of them; he lives only in the "now." May's kind and soothing voice and her patience, along with her affectionate touch, soothed Leo. Clearly, there was a strong connecting and connection between the two of them as there is with many persons with dementia and their families.

After connection, Waldfogel's (1997) second identified element of spirituality is meaning and purpose in life. The emphasis here is on coherence and continuity. According to Waldfogel, "the recovery of meaning in illness and of coherence in one's personal narrative appear to be central to the healing process" (p. 965). Post (1998), in discussing Willem de Kooning, the famous abstract expressionist painter and his struggle with Alzheimer's Disease, summarizes the art critic Kay Larson (1997). According to Larson, to suggest that de Kooning needed his disease to free himself would be unkind. Nonetheless, the violence done to him by Alzheimer's could not stop the effects of a lifetime of disci-

pline and love of painting. When Alzheimer's struck, the artist was prepared. If he was unaware of what he was doing, maybe it didn't matter
to him because his love of work sustained him.

This brief excerpt illustrates several points: (a) Alzheimer's Disease
is an equalizer—it strikes both the famous and the unknown; (b) habits
acquired over a lifetime are always becoming; (c) Alzheimer's Disease
does not necessarily erode emotion or passion for what one loves; and
(d) what one loves can sustain a person through Alzheimer's Disease.
Above all, the excerpt about de Kooning illustrates the connection between the artist and his work and how coherence and continuity provided meaning and purpose in his life.

Waldfogel's (1997) third identified element of spirituality is transcendence. Transcendence is usually associated with transformative life
experiences. These experiences often elevate individuals to a higher
level of humanness by extending their sense of reality to what was previously unknown to them or, in persons with Alzheimer's Disease, to what
was once known to them but now forgotten.

Although it is not always so, some experiences of transcendence have
a spiritual dimension and meaning, which might be described as seeking
the sacred in life. We have read accounts of persons rendered mute by
advanced dementia who, after seeing or hearing something that touched
them deeply, begin to hum, sing, cry, sob, and cease wandering. They
often surprised both their families and their healthcare providers who
believed that long ago they had experienced "loss of self." From a phenomenological viewpoint, however, the behaviors are not surprising.
These severely demented persons were living fully their possibilities.
The message here is this: No matter how demented individuals appear,
families and healthcare providers can never assume a loss of humanness.
Persons with severe dementia "are becoming." To exclude or diminish
their "becoming" is to do violence to their humanness and to do harm
to them in the name of a particular interpretation of quality of life.

Here are excerpts from a story that also addresses transcendence.
Jan, in her mid-40s, exhibited symptoms of Alzheimer's Disease. Jan
speaks to us about her disease:

Dementia is the disease, they say, cause unknown. At this point it no longer
mattered to me just what that cause was because the tests eliminated the revers-
ible ones, my hospital coverage was gone, and my spirit was too worn to even
care about the name of something irreversible. . . .

I was angry, I was broken and this was something I could not fix, nor to date can anyone fix it for me. How was I to live without myself? I wanted Jan back. . . .

An intense fear enveloped my entire being as I mourned the loss of what was and the hopes and dreams that might never be. How could this be happening to me? What exactly will become of me? These questions occupied much of my time for far too many days.

Then one day as I fumbled around the kitchen to prepare a pot of coffee, something caught my eye through the window. It had snowed and I had truly forgotten what a beautiful sight a soft, gentle snowfall could be. . . . As I bent down to gather a mass of those radiantly white flakes . . . it seemed as though I could do nothing but marvel at their beauty. . . .

Later I realized . . . [that I was able to see] a snowfall through the same innocent eyes of the child I once was, so many years ago. I am still here, I thought, and there will be wonders to be held in each new day; they are just different now. (Post, 1995, p. 19)

Jan's story speaks eloquently to living fully in the possibilities. At first angered and broken by her diagnosis of Alzheimer's Disease, she was able to transcend the disease after an encounter with a beautiful snowfall that left her revering the awesomeness of nature. Jan had not stopped becoming but was able to see her life through each new day's wonders. The disease was the same but Jan was not; her becoming allowed her to value each day greatly but in a different way. She had rediscovered the sacred in her life that she had known as a child.

Enhancing the Experience of Spirituality for Persons With Dementia and Their Healthcare Providers

One of the premises of this chapter is that healthcare providers have a moral obligation to rethink the assumptions that underlie quality of life for persons with dementia and their families. We have argued that individuals with dementia, no matter how severe, have the moral status of persons. We also believe that enhancing spirituality improves a person's quality of life; therefore, we urge nurses and other healthcare providers, within the scope of their practice, to attend to the spiritual needs of patients in addition to other healthcare practices that enhance quality of life.

Howe (1998) believes that healthcare providers' attitudes can diminish quality of life in persons with dementia. He discusses how healthcare providers' negative emotions (i.e., irrational anger, guilt, glee) can harm patients. To overcome the problem of healthcare providers who do not feel loving toward persons with dementia, he suggests that they work with carers who do genuinely love these persons. Howe (1998) concludes by saying, "if care providers only love these patients just enough to try to help them, this could be more than enough" (p. 8).

Long (1997) also focuses on carers, but her emphasis is specifically on the nurse and spirituality. She believes that nurses must know how to care for themselves in all dimensions, including the spiritual dimension, before they can care for others. This spiritual becoming begins with a relationship with the self. Long then goes on to help nurses explore a spiritual journey of becoming through the following:

1. *"The Spiritual Dimension of Self"* (Long, 1997, pp. 499–500)—The journey toward the spiritual dimension of self takes the nurse to the innermost self—a place of solitude where the nurse is connected with his or her unique "oneness" and how that oneness that is the nurse relates to and affects others.
2. *"Touching the Untouchable and Clasping the Unseen"* (Long, 1997, p. 500)—Nurses can connect with unseen persons' spirituality through empathy. For example, in the writing of this chapter, the authors were deeply moved by some of the harms experienced by persons with dementia; we were also moved by these persons' gallant struggles to transcend their illnesses. We also had a desire to right the wrongs done to the humanness of individuals with dementia and to reach out and touch those who were seemingly unseen because of severe dementia.
3. *"Embracing the Essence of Humanness"* (Long, 1997, p. 500)—Long views the essence of humanness as the spiritual part of the self. The crux of embracing the essence of humanness is for the nurse to allow all individuals to express their spirituality and/or religiosity in their own ways and without judgment or intrusions by the nurse. To do less is to diminish their humanness.
4. *"Personal Spiritual Pain"* (Long, 1997, p. 500)—According to Long, often personal spiritual pain is greatest when the nurse is facing a major personal crisis. A part of the personal spiritual pain associated with the crisis is a loneliness of spirit that can affect nursing care. For example, a nurse working on an Alzheimer's unit at the same time that the nurse's mother is diagnosed with the disease may experience spiritual pain. This situation may be so close to home that the nurse begins to distance her- or himself from those persons with dementia who desperately need love and care. At this moment the nurse is unable to live fully in the possibilities.

5. *"Embracing Loneliness and Emptiness"* (Long, 1997, p. 503)—If spirituality and wholeness are interrelated, and the authors believe that they are, then nurses will experience all emotions, including painful ones such as loneliness and emptiness. According to Long (1997), it is through embracing loneliness and emptiness as part of oneself that caring occurs; this caring allows nurses to be in tune with and tolerant of other persons, even when they annoy or displease us. Certainly, some behaviors of persons with Alzheimer's Disease could be viewed as annoying or displeasing, but nurses who have embraced their own loneliness and emptiness will recognize it in their patients and view these persons with compassion instead of unkindness.

6. *"Slipping and Sliding"* (Long, 1997, p. 503)—According to Long, "The dual capacity to feel true to self and to take self for granted slips and slides in most people's lives . . ." (p. 503). The need and goal for nurses are to feel inwardly safe, secure, and worthy. These traits are related to "being spiritual" (p. 503) and are considered essential to the relationship part of nursing. To preserve humanness and enhance spiritual becoming of persons with dementia, healthcare providers must be aware of their interpersonal practices. Kitwood (1998) has identified 10 such positive interpersonal practices: recognition, negotiation, collaboration, play, timalation [massage], celebration, relaxation, validation, holding, and facilitation. In addition Kitwood (1997) notes that research has indicated that the psychological environment can affect neuronal growth or, put another way, "that care practices can have neurological consequences" (p. 63). By following excellence of practice, the authors believe that spiritual experience and quality of life are enhanced for both persons with dementia and their healthcare providers.

In part 3, we have argued for the moral status of individuals with dementia; we have examined the link between humanness and spirituality; we have argued that attending to spirituality can enhance the quality of life of individuals with dementia; and we have examined how healthcare providers, in their practice, can enhance a patient's experience of spirituality.

A Call to Thinking

In this chapter we have examined the danger to patients when quality of life judgments follow too rigidly from the biomedical model of medicine. We argued for a broader interpretation of health and illness grounded in interpretive phenomenology. We leave you with the following thoughts:

- The biomedical model of medicine has influenced interpretations of quality of life that may lead to oppressing patients. How can healthcare workers contribute to a more inclusive model of medicine? How can broader definitions of quality of life be developed?
- Evidence from patient and family perspectives show the ineffectiveness of the biomedical model to determine the quality of life of persons with dementia. What kind of model is required to ensure an interpretation of quality of life that is open to the full range of possibilities of persons with dementia?
- The unique perspective of persons with dementia can only be fully appreciated through an understanding of life narratives that healthcare professionals should use to make decisions respecting patients' values. How can healthcare providers remain open to valuing persons with dementia? How can healthcare providers come to know the life narratives of persons with dementia?
- Recognizing the humanness of individuals experiencing dementia, despite the loss of cognitive functions, helps to limit their exposure to oppressive treatment. How does an exclusive appeal to the criterion of cognitive functioning contribute to oppressing persons with dementia? How can other qualities, including spirituality, help us to appreciate the humanness of persons with dementia?

Nothing that we have said in this chapter should be construed as denying to healthcare professionals the obligation to make sound medical judgments about treatment. We acknowledge and support the need for professional judgments that therapeutic interventions may be futile, in the sense of not able to achieve their medical objectives, or, worse, pointlessly prolonging the dying process. Further, we agree that quality of life is an important consideration in determining treatment options for individuals; however, we have argued that the appeal to quality of life does not introduce the element of objectivity that early proponents believed. Quality of life judgments are perspectival; our position is that the primary perspective should be that of the patient.

In some cases achieving the patient's perspective can be difficult. It is certainly difficult in the advanced stages of chronic conditions like Alzheimer's Disease. For this reason we believe that preparation for quality-of-life decisions must begin long before the final stages make such inquiries impossible. Therefore, healthcare providers have a moral obligation to establish, whenever possible, narrative histories of the patients under their care. Failure to do so may result in harming patients in the name of quality of life.

References

Aiken, W. (1982). The quality of life. *Applied Philosophy, 1*, 26–36.

Bayley, J. (1999). *Elegy for Iris.* New York: Picador USA.

Brody, H. (1987). *Stories of sickness.* New Haven, CT: Yale University Press.

Carlberg, A. (1998). *The moral Rubicon: A study of the principles of sanctity of life and quality of life in bioethics.* Lund, Sweden: Lund University Press.

Cassell, E. J. (1993). The sorcerer's broom: Medicine's rampant technology. *Hastings Center Report, 23*(6), 32–39.

Coles, R. (1989). *The call of stories: Teaching and the moral imagination.* Boston: Houghton Mifflin.

Congdon, J., & Magilvy, J. (1998). Rural nursing homes: A housing option for older adults. *Geriatric Nursing, 19*(3), 157–159.

Cox, C. (1986). The interaction model of client health behavior: Application to the study of community based elders. *Advances in Nursing Science, 9*(1), 40–57.

Edgar, E. (1998). Quality of life indicators. *Encyclopedia of Applied Ethics* (Vol. 3, pp. 759–776). San Diego, CA: Academic Press.

Emblen, J. D. (1992). *Religion* and *Spirituality* defined according to current use in nursing literature. *Journal of Professional Nursing, 8*, 41–47.

Estes, C. L. (1979). *The aging enterprise.* San Francisco: Jossey-Bass.

Estes, C. L., & Binney, E. A. (1989). The biomedicalization of aging: Dangers and dilemmas. *The Gerontologist, 29*(5), 587–596.

Ferenz, L. D. (2000). The aesthetics of dementia care: Some final thoughts from Tom Kitwood. *The Journal of Clinical Ethics, 11*(1), 69–72.

Ferrucci, L., Guralnik, J., Pahor, M. Corti, M., & Havlik, R. (1997). Hospital diagnoses, Medicare charges, and nursing home admissions in the year when older persons become disabled. *JAMA, 277*(9), 728–734.

Fiumara, G. C. (1990). *The other side of language: A philosophy of listening.* New York: Routledge.

Fletcher, J. (1972). Indicators of humanhood: A tentative profile of man. *Hastings Center Report, 2*(6), 1–4.

Fletcher, J. (1974). Four indicators of humanhood—the enquiry matures. *Hastings Center Report, 4*(6), 4–7.

Fletcher, J. (1975). The "right" to live and the "right" to die. In M. Kohl (Ed.), *Beneficent euthanasia* (pp. 44–53). Buffalo, NY: Prometheus Books.

Foucault, M. (1973). *The birth of the clinic: An archeology of the human sciences.* New York: Vintage Press.

Gill, T. M., & Feinstein, A. R. (1994). A critical appraisal of the quality of quality of life measurements. *JAMA, 272*(8), 619–626.

Goldberg, B. (1998). Connection: An exploration of spirituality in nursing care. *Journal of Advanced Nursing, 27*, 836–842.

Goodinson, S. M., & Singleton, J. (1989). Quality of life: A critical review of current concepts, measures and their clinical implications. *International Journal of Nursing Studies, 26*(4), 327–341.

Habermas, J. (1984) The theory of communicative action. *Reason and the rationalisation of society* (Vol. 1, T. McCarthy, Trans.). Boston: Beacon Press.

Hahn, R. A. (1995). *Sickness and healing. An anthropological perspective.* New Haven and London: Yale University Press.

Heidegger, M. (1971). *Poetry language thought* (A. Hofstadter, Trans.). New York: Harper & Row.

Heidegger, M. (1977) What calls for thinking? In D. Krell (Ed.), *Basic writings* (pp. 369–391). New York: HarperCollins.

Hiatt, J. F. (1986). Spirituality, medicine, and healing. *Southern Medical Journal, 79*(6), 736–743.

Holstein, M. B. (1998). Ethics and Alzheimer's Disease: Widening the lens. *The Journal of Clinical Ethics, 9*(1), 13–22.

Howe, E. G. (1998). Caring for patients with dementia: An indication for "emotional communism." *The Journal of Clinical Ethics, 9*(1), 3–11.

Kapp, M. B. (1998). Persons with dementia as "liability magnets": Ethical implications. *The Journal of Clinical Ethics, 9*(1), 66–70.

Karnofsky, D., & Burchenal, J. (1949). The clinical evaluation of chemotherapeutic agents in cancer. In C. M. Maclead (Ed.), *Evaluation of chemotherapeutic agents* (pp. 191–205). New York: Columbia Press.

Keyserlingk, E. W. (1997). Quality of life decisions and the hopelessly ill patient: The physician as moral agent and truth teller. In K. Hoshino (Ed.), *Japanese and Western bioethics* (pp. 103–116). Amsterdam: Kluwer Academic Publishers.

Kitwood, T. (1997). *Dementia reconsidered: The person comes first.* Buckingham: Open University Press.

Kitwood, T. (1998). Toward a theory of dementia care: Ethics and interaction. *The Journal of Clinical Inquiry, 9*(1), 23–34.

LaPuma, J., & Lawlor, E. F. (1990). Quality adjusted life years: Ethical implications for physicians and policymakers. *JAMA, 263*(21), 2917–2921.

Larson, K. (1997). Willem de Kooning and Alzheimer's. *World & I, 12*(7), 297–299.

Lauver, D. R. (2000). Commonalities in women's spirituality and women's health. *Advances in Nursing Science, 22*(3), 76–88.

Leplege, A., & Hunt, S. (1997). The problem of quality of life in medicine. *JAMA, 278*(1), 47–50.

Long, A. (1997). Nursing: A spiritual perspective. *Nursing Ethics: An International Journal for Healthcare Professionals, 4,* 496–510.

Luborsky, M. (1994). The cultural adversity of physical disability: Erosion of full adult personhood. *Journal of Aging Studies, 8,* 239–253.

Lyman, K. A. (1998). Living with Alzheimer's Disease: The creation of meaning among persons with dementia. *The Journal of Clinical Ethics, 9*(1), 49–57.

McCormick, R. A. (1974). To save or let die. *America, 131*(1), 6–10.

McCurdy, D. B. (1998). Personhood, spirituality, and hope in the care of human beings with dementia. *The Journal of Clinical Ethics, 9*(1), 81–91.

McSherry, W., & Draper, P. (1998). The debates emerging from the literature surrounding the concept of spirituality as applied to nursing. *Journal of Advanced Nursing, 27,* 683–691.

Moody, H. R. (1992). *Ethics in an aging society.* Baltimore: The Johns Hopkins University Press.

Musschenga, A. W. (1997). The relation between concepts of quality of life, health and happiness. *The Journal of Medicine and Philosophy, 22,* 11–28.

Nelson, J. L. (1998). Reasons and feelings, duty and dementia. *The Journal of Clinical Ethics, 9*(1) 58–65.

Post, S. G. (1995). *The moral challenge of Alzheimer's Disease.* Baltimore: The Johns Hopkins University Press.

Post, S. G. (1998). The fears of forgetfulness: A grassroots approach to an ethics of Alzheimer's Disease. *The Journal of Clinical Ethics, 9*(1), 71–80.

Post, S. G., & Whitehouse, P. J. (1995). Fairhill guidelines on ethics of the care of people with Alzheimer's Disease: A clinical summary. *JAGS, 43,* 1423–1429.

Reich, W. T. (1978). Quality of life. *Encyclopedia of Bioethics* (Vol. 2, pp. 829–840). New York: The Free Press.

Rich, B. A. (1996). The values history: Restoring narrative identity to long term care. *Journal of Ethics, Law, and Aging, 2*(2), 75–84.

Russell, C. (1996). Passion and heretics: Meaning in life and quality of life of persons with dementia. *The Journal of the American Geriatrics Society, 44*(11), 1400–1402.

Sabat, S. R. (1998). Voices of Alzheimer's Disease sufferers: A call for treatment based on personhood. *The Journal of Clinical Ethics, 9*(1), 35–48.

Sacks, O. D. (1985). *The man who mistook his wife for a hat: And other clinical tales.* New York: Simon & Schuster.

Shelp, E. E. (1986). *Born to die? Deciding the fate of critically ill newborns.* New York: Free Press.

Sorrell, J. M. (2000). Ethical concerns of caring for patients with Alzheimer's Disease. Unpublished research.

Spitzer, W. O., Dobson, A. J., Hall, J., Chesterman E., & Levi, J. (1981). Measuring the quality of life of cancer patients. *Journal of Chronic Disease, 34,* 585–597.

Starr, T. J., Pearlman, R. A., & Uhlmann, R. F. (1986). Quality of life and resuscitation decisions in elderly patients. *Journal of General Internal Medicine, 1,* 373–379.

Stein, H. F. (1990). *American medicine as culture.* Boulder, CO: Westview Press.

Stoll, B. (1977). *Breast cancer management—early and late.* London: Heinemann.

Veatch, R. M. (1993). The impending collapse of the whole-brain definition of death. *Hastings Center Report, 23*(4), 18–24.

Waldfogel, S. (1997). Spirituality in medicine. *Complementary and Alternative Therapies in Primary Care, 24,* 963–976.

Walter, J. J. (1988). The meaning and validity of quality of life judgments in contemporary Roman Catholic medical ethics. *Louvain Studies, 13,* 195–208.

Walter, J. J. (1995). Quality of life in clinical decisions. *Encyclopedia of Bioethics* (Rev. ed., Vol. 2, pp. 1352–1358). New York: Simon and Schuster Macmillan.

Young, K. J., & Longman, A. J. (1983). Quality of life and persons with melanoma: A pilot study. *Cancer Nursing, 6,* 219–225.

2

Neither Here Nor There

The Story of a Health Professional's Experience With Getting Care and Needing Caring

Kathryn Hopkins Kavanagh

Prologue

This interpretive study revolves around the story of a critical care nurse who, in her early forties and midcareer, developed end stage renal disease. For nearly 8 months following renal and pancreatic transplantation, Carol Ann Rooks repeatedly required intensive medical and nursing care. It was a time of struggling for connections and fearing gaps, of needing vigilance and apprehending powerlessness, of longing to be cared for (that is, being the object of caretaking practices) and for caring (experiencing meaningful connecting and feeling cared about).

As Carol Ann groped her way through a fearful abyss of catastrophic illness, she sought the meaning of caring and its practices, when what really mattered was often unclear to others. This essay emphasizes that care and caring in the clearing where what is known to patients (pain, vulnerability, vigilance) became known to Carol Ann as a patient as well as a nurse. It is, in short, about narrowing the gap between critical illness as it is understood by those experiencing it and the meaning of critical illness for those who care for patients.

Carol Ann's search for meaning led to an understanding of critical illness for both patients and caring nonpatients as merely different facets of the same phenomenon. When that sharing and connecting fails, when patients and clinicians are strangers at the deepest levels of human familiarity, the patient is left to flounder, not necessarily without care but without caring. Carol Ann often said that when she returned to nursing, she would be, after her experience as a patient and stepping through the looking glass into a world unlike any expected, a different nurse than she was before. Although Carol Ann will not return to nursing, her story can.

Carol Ann approached the transplant with a health professional's knowledge tempered by a patient's optimism.

I don't know what I anticipated when I said, "Yea, let's go for a kidney." Somehow I thought it would be zip-zap and it would be done. It didn't work out that way. . . .

There are a lot of things that I do remember and a lot of things that I don't remember about what happened to me. Some have been blurred by drugs. I clearly remember hallucinating when I first came out of kidney surgery. I remember my father telling me that the surgery was over and that I had a new kidney. I had realized neither. I kept hearing nurses' voices saying things about intubating patients, and all night long I feared that I would be nasally intubated.

That was the beginning. Carol Ann decided to chronicle her story after the transplanted pancreas, transplanted with the kidney, failed and was removed. Narratives about the lived experiences of patients who have endured the surgery and subsequent treatment regimens of transplant are rare in the literature. On the other hand, even scarcer is the experiential account of a patient who, as a healthcare provider, understands the meanings of transplantation from both perspectives.

Carol Ann found herself thrust into a maze of anti-rejection drugs, antibiotics, exploratory laparotomies, infection caused by a bowel perforation that resulted in four additional major surgeries, a temporary ileostomy, a lengthy series of additional infections, severe malnutrition and total parenteral nutrition, a liver biopsy, numerous kidney biopsies, reanastomosis of the bowel, and multiple hemorrhages and blood transfusions. All of these well-intended invasions of her life preceded her discharge home, 8 months and five major surgeries *after* the transplant. Discharge meant a new profusion of self-care medications, equipment, and lifestyle changes. The care she received both helped and hindered Carol Ann's prolonged and painful passage.

The Approach

Interpretation, Clinical Ethnography, Phenomenology, and Narrative

The phenomena of our inquiry, care and caring, are deeply embedded in American culture (Denzin, 1997; Kleinman, 1995) and its reflections in the subcultures of nursing and medicine (Lupton, 1994; Stein, 1990). The concern of medical anthropology with "culture, science, knowledge, medicine, bodies and discourses" (Tomlinson, 1999, p. 8) makes its biocultural approach (Morris, 1998) highly apropos to nursing and medical practice. Furthermore, anthropology's emphasis on interrelationships between ethics and context make it a particularly fitting partner for nursing's shift from an epistemological focus on patterns of knowing to ontological reflections on ways of being (Silva, Sorrell, & Sorrell, 1995).

Traditionally concerned with the interpretation and lived experience of illness (Lupton, 1994), medical anthropology generally explores the ethos of care and reality of cost (in its many forms) in the theater of practice. Emphasizing the experience of persons in the situation, illness narratives (Kleinman, 1988a; Morse & Johnson, 1991) provide a medium for that exploration through personalized, Gestalt-like perspectives that counter the problem of limiting meaning of experience to theoretical discussion (Benner, 1984; Steeves, 1992). Illness narratives provide situated discourses—real life stories—in the language of those who live them. Their very reflectivity allows meaning to reveal itself through the telling and retelling that lays bare images in deeper layers, perspectives, colors, and shades.

Given that "the very nature of the human realm is interpretive" (Hultgren, 1994, p. 25), hermeneutic phenomenology is the study of the lifeworld that we experience immediately as reality (Husserl, 1970). Hermeneutics, as an art of interpretation, conceives of the entire phenomenon as not a simple substance but as a complex system more rooted in culture than the natural sciences (Honderich, 1995; Palmer, 1969). Recollective, thoughtful, and mindful (van Manen, 1990), phenomenology focuses on lived experience as we live pre-reflexively through it, rather than as we conceptualize, categorize, or reflect on it.

Sometimes, however, philosophies and research approaches—being part and parcel of the world and not transcendent views somehow beyond that (Jackson, 1996)—are most effectively brought together in efforts to understand complex phenomena of human living. The domain of phenomenology, being-in-the-world, cannot be wholly construed in terms of "self-enclosed features of human subjectivity" (Casey, 1991, p. xix; Jackson, 1996, p. 1). Because interpretative practice is mediated by discourse that constitutes distinct, albeit overlapping, realities (Gubrium & Holstein, 2000), understanding prospers through reflective and contextual enrichment. Interpretive practice is not socially arbitrary; it is variegated and shared while being biographically and situationally informed.

One of myriad approaches to managing the complexity and fluidity of real life phenomena is to exercise various genres of ethnography (Tedlock, 2000) in conjunction with phenomenology. Long used to shape narrative with representations—ethnicity, gender, occupational vantage, age, and innumerable others—in time and place, ethnography fashions cultural understandings through kaleidoscopes of intertwining voices (Ellis & Bochner, 1996). While hermeneutic phenomenology provides a central framing for seeing the possibilities available to understanding the self and its world, it lends itself graciously to affiliation with ethnography's even more broadly contextualized, multileveled frame of reference. It is the purview of critical ethnography, for example, to question how those phenomena come to be what they are and to function as they do (Street, 1992) and that of interpretive ethnography to closely examine phenomena that function meaningfully in the culture of a given society (Denzin, 1997; Knaack, 1984; Kockelmans, 1975; Richardson & Fowers, 1998a, b). Without restriction to a structured methodology, the intent of interpretive ethnography is to examine the transaction between the situation and the person who experiences it in ways that help clarify personal and social meanings within the historical and cultural situation.

Understanding what the world we experience and live in is *about* helps explicate relationships of the whole with both reasoning and feeling. The intention is to grasp, in creating the evidence that is interpreted, the inner essential nature—the true being—of a thing. Synchronized phenomenological and ethnographic interpretative understandings (*Verstehen*) meld hermeneutic ways of explicating a phenomenon, making it both maximally reasonable and human in familiar ways (Heidegger, 1962; Koch, 1995; Kockelmans, 1975; Leonard, 1989) and contextualizing it in the community and time, as well as the lived experience, of the real world. The interpretive, contextual, and critical stances become one, emerging with the telling of the story and relating its meanings through ongoing cycles of sharing, discourse, and reinterpretation.

The confluence of phenomenology and ethnography wreathes the theory of the social with that of writing so that the social locates itself within a text (Derrida, 1981). Healthcare always implicates an ethical as well as spatial and temporal dimension. Carol Ann's story, being no exception, provides a thick description of medical ethics (D. Davis, 1991). This contextualized recreation of the world accommodates new technologies, shifting systems, paradigmatic revolutions, and a poststructuralist world no longer conforming to singular journeys along recognizable paths. In other words, understanding phenomena and what the world we experience and live in is *about* is served through creation of a context with boundaries so that the narrative of self can support an emancipatory, interpretive interactionism that extends beyond given phenomena (Denzin, 1997). While ethnography brings to the forefront varying relationships between sickness and healing as they are culturally expressed in changing historical contingencies (Fábrega, 1997), phenomenology brings us to meaning as it is lived. Interpretive ethnography helps make sense of, reveal the meaning of, that being. Thus, text and context are embedded together in historicity and contingency that demand to be reckoned with in a realist epistemology. Together these perspectives can ask the paramount existential question: "How is this, or is this not, a healing experience?"

Clinical ethnography engages interpretive phenomenology in the study of illness experience to uncover practical experiential knowledge gained by patients (Doolittle, 1994). Since all disease and illness are experienced and interpreted, the recovery of the social body involves a body engaged in meaningful activity while simultaneously suffering losses and changes, often resulting in a focus on its parts rather than the whole. While things show up that matter (Dreyfus, 1987), what *matters* may be uneven or unclear (Merleau-Ponty, 1962). In that light, the contextualization of ethnography, in partnership with the hermeneutic understanding of phenomenology, is preferable to either approach alone in embracing the experiences of individuals and interpreting them in their constitutively cultural worlds. Although it might be argued that phenomenology alone may be so inclusive, the first author's orientation to anthropology fosters a bias toward the marriage of the two interpretive approaches to inquiry.

In sum, meaning, coming as much from within experience as given to it, is revealed through interpretation or hermeneutical reflection. Phenomenological interpretation depends on sharing the interpretive act through the availability of descriptive narrative from the individual experiencing the phenomenon. Whereas narrative represents an individual conversing with him- or herself, empathy allows sharing of that by orienting another to the participant's experience and meaning-making (Baillie, 1996; Josselson & Lieblich, 1995). Discovery comes about when narrative, within the totality of its text and context, encounters an empathic stance fostering "vicarious introspection" (Kohut, 1977, p. 306). In healthcare, such findings have potential to relate directly to understanding and transforming practice (Diekelmann, 1991). That potential is enhanced by bringing the interpretive perspective of phenomenology together with the traditionally more critical stance of clinically situated ethnography.

Caring

As the expressive art of being fully present to another person, caring takes on fundamental importance in situations involving serious illness (A. J. Davis, 1981). Encompassing components of activity and attitude (Griffin, 1983), caring can be usefully differentiated into the more abstract caring *about* and relatively direct caring *for* (Jecker & Self, 1991; Watson, 1985), as well as into diverse traits, functions, and types (Chesla, 1994; Morse, Bottorff, Neander, & Solberg, 1991; Morse, Solberg, Neander, Bottorff, & Johnson, 1990), and relationships with psychological, social, and ethical orientations (Fry, 1989; Puka, 1990). The preeminence of caring in nursing practice is a major concern when norms for practice reflect cultural values that are more individualistic and materialistic than humanistic and relational (Benner, Tanner, & Chesla, 1996; Benner & Wrubel, 1989; Forrest, 1989; Hanneman, 1996).

Ideologically, nursing struggles to promote caring in the sense of enabling connecting and concern (Dreyfus, Dreyfus, & Athanasiou, 1986) as those are affiliated with needs focusing on the integrity of the person (Holmes & Warelow, 1997) and commitment to the alleviation of vulnerability (Gadow, 1988). Nonetheless, in critical care practice settings, where "bio-power" reflects deep political, economic, and cultural processes (Foucault, 1973, p. 199), human connections and communication can be compromised by orientations to machines, invasion of personal space, objectification of persons in patient roles, and environmental imbalances leading to sensory overload or deprivation (De-Visser, 1981; Gadow, 1989; Halm & Alpen, 1993). Research in critical care settings attests to nurses' frustration with their limited roles in patient care, considerable confusion around what is the most appropriate care, and the inability of some critical care settings to foster the caring and compassion that many acutely ill patients need (Asch, Shea, Jedrziewski, & Bosk, 1997).

Allied with concern about the sparse attention conferred upon caring in nursing school curricula (Cooper, 1991; Gunby, 1996) is a pronounced interest in recognition and development of caring as integral to expert clinical nursing practice (Benner, 1984; Benner, Tanner, & Chesla, 1996; Diekelmann, 1991; Riley & Omery, 1996). Immediately relevant to Carol Ann's story is Drew's (1986) research distinguishing specific power-centered practices that depersonalize and exclude from those that authenticate patients. Similarly germane is Minick's (1995) study with critical care nurses, which demonstrates the benefits gained by nurses' involvement with patients in terms of assessments leading to early recognition of problems with vulnerable patients' illness situations.

Although constituent details of expert and nonexpert practice are difficult to articulate, Hanneman (1996) provides a grounded theory that depicts patterns of expert caring practice characterized by regard for patient response and outcomes and by presence within a patient situation, that is, an unimpaired sense of "being there." Such attending presence has also been described as attunement to the reality of a situation (Griffin, 1983) and willingness to engage, support, and learn from one another (Cooper, 1991). In expert caring (Benner, Tanner, & Chesla, 1996), clinical judgment and attention to the interactive situation are equally important. Using technology and technologically derived data to help *humanize* practice, caring in expert practice is replete with focused assessments, awareness of the interrelatedness and possibilities of situations, and decisive action guided by a strong orientation to patient-outcome and minimal occupation with skills (Hanneman, 1996). Caring involves, in other words, a professional artistry (Schon, 1991) fabricated of knowing, prioritizing, and forgetting that allows using artifacts in praxis so that thoughtful action renders technology the important but secondary status of a tool employed to reveal other realms of meaning and nature (Sandelowski, 1997).

Benner, Hooper-Kyriakidis, and Stannard (1999) build on previous studies of reflective practice to delineate the nature of ethical clinical reasoning as response-based and proactive, sensitive to continuous situational change, and particular to specific patients and their significant others. The caring clinician, situated to facilitate learning the immediate situation and needs, engages in practical and ongoing dialogue with all aspects of that situation through a perpetual acuity that is linked to emotional engagement with both the problem and the interpersonal situation (Benner, Hooper-Kyriakidis, & Stannard, 1999; Benner & Wrubel, 1989). This clinical reasoning stance becomes, in essence, the integral constituent of praxis (the working out of knowledge, inquiry, relationships, and action in place) and of agency (the ability to influence the situation [Benner, Tanner, & Chesla, 1996]). Together, praxis and agency allow effective, quality care and management of breakdowns.

Can and does this actually occur in healthcare situations, and how is such caring experienced? Embodied understandings in taken-for-granted, highly skilled responses elude ready explication, although interpretive inquiry makes possible their meaningful exploration (Benner & Wrubel, 1989). That is the purpose of this chapter. It is Carol Ann's and my conclusion that, for a healing experience to occur, care must involve adequate expertise to allow technology to safely take a secondary status and thus make room for the ethical clinical reasoning that promotes *caring*.

The Way of Inquiry

Interpretive inquiry turns to emergent designs to emphasize the complexity of human life in efforts to apprehend meanings in occurrences as they are contextualized in given times and places. In this study, inquiry proceeded pragmatically with both of us participating in ongoing discourse, interpreting that discourse, and incorporating the interpretations into understandings of the continuing and ever-changing situation (Steeves & Kahn, 1995). These cyclical strategies created a milieu for and way of revealing socially embedded knowledge (Benner & Wrubel, 1989; Kleinman, 1995) found in Carol Ann's story. In other words, interrelated reflections lead to the very process that Frank (1995) develops in *The Wounded Storyteller*, that is, thinking with stories. While interpreting clinical stories nurtures focus on the "therapeutic emplotment" (Mattingly, 1994) that shapes clients', physicians', and other healthcare providers' encounters in clinical contexts, broader biocultural understandings (Morris, 1998) support critique of the professional artistry (Schon, 1991), crafting of therapeutics and care, and formulation of what it is that "we think medicine should care about" (B. J. Good, 1994, p. 199).

In exposing social narrative and analyzing medical encounters, a relational posture is revealed that critiques ethical narratives between individuals, perhaps especially women, and their caretakers (Boykin & Schoenhofer, 1991; K. Davis, 1993; Fisher, 1986; Gadow, 1994; Martin, 1987). While narrative allows a strong and oriented relation to be maintained with a phenomenon (van Manen, 1990), emotional and physical turmoil associated with painful experience can intercept memory and recollection (Hollway & Jefferson, 1997; Schutze, 1992), thus requiring marked endurance to create the text (that is, the narrative description of the experience with the phenomenon) that serves as the object of interpretation (Allen & Jensen, 1990).

To grasp the meaning of the care that Carol Ann experienced and the caring that she needed, we recorded her story during several dozen (close to 100) sessions. Our communicative alliance encompassed interviewing (truly *inter-views* [Kvale, 1996]), conversing, engaged dialogue, and much active listening to shape the telling of the story and to get to the larger, contextual ethnographic narrative (as it would be a different story in a different context), for sets of relationships between actions and accounts are complex (P. Atkinson, 1995).

Although clinical exchanges and much of clinical work is accomplished through talk, it is hardly reducible to conversation alone (P. Atkinson, 1995). I (Kathy) created and maintained extensive field notes and transcribed audiotapes (Lapadat & Lindsay, 1999) with Carol Ann's evolving story, with copies of the entire documentation shared with Carol Ann on a continual basis—even when she was too ill to do more than know they were there. Since the account that is read rarely, if ever, leaves as clear a picture as the account that is heard, attending to the narrative, both oral and written, allowed us to search for the unity of the themes and plot, its logic as a product of culture, its aesthetic–spiritual and historical foundations, and the inherent struggle for existence (Linde, 1993; Olrik, 1992). Forming a variant of an insider/outsider research team (Barry, Britten, Barber, Bradley, & Stevenson, 1999; Bartunek & Louis, 1996; Richards, 1999), we depended on the extensive recordings to chronicle, as well as to spotlight, Carol Ann's experience as a case study for distillation and interpretation of caring and care as parts of human culture and experience (Baer, 1987; Feagin, Orum, & Sjoberg, 1991; Stein, 1995).

Since Carol Ann was a former student and teaching assistant of mine, we knew each other well and shared a continuing friendship and collegial relationship. That formed a natural basis of concern and mutuality, allowing for reciprocity as nurses and coresearchers (Campbell & Bunting, 1991; Harris, Ryan, & Belmont, 1997). Our conversing was flexible, often drifting comfortably into topics peripheral to the task. Although our relationship and use of self threatened to limit our range of interpretations, it inhibited ambiguity as well, and ethical issues could be promptly resolved in favor of advocacy over the research imperative (Rew, Bechtal, & Sapp, 1993).

In short, the essential purpose for being together was visiting rather than research, although visiting has been proposed as an alternative research method (Running, 1994) and served as such for us. This usually took place in early evenings while Carol Ann was hospitalized and midmornings after her discharge. My evening visits meant missing most of the daytime interactions, both careful and careless, which encouraged Carol Ann's descriptions of those encounters. Telling and retelling her lived experiences prompted multiple layers of continuous deliberation, interpretation, and reinterpretation on both our parts. At other times, our time was spent together in simple restful quietude when Carol Ann was too sick or too exhausted for active dialogue. Although visiting can be a format for interviewing techniques (Athay 1993; Burgoon, Olney, & Coker, 1987; Meeker, 1984; Rank & LeCroy, 1983; Running, 1996), as well as a medium for social exchange and creating collaborative relationships or performing specific tasks (Aaronson, 1989; Barkauskas, 1983; Halpern, 1984; Hancock & Pelton, 1989; Keller, Flatten, & Wilhite, 1988; Leitko & Peterson, 1982; Lomnitz, 1988; Scott, 1992; Warry, 1992), our visiting was founded primarily in concern (Joel, 1997), hope for healing (Weibel-Orlando, 1989), and friendship (Harris, Ryan, & Belmont, 1997).

We often pondered the question of the impact our inquiry had on Carol Ann's recovery (Barry et al., 1999; Kleinman, 1988a; Kvale, 1999), particularly when our visits and discussions led to explicating the unclear, even the unthought. It is well known that, in itself, telling stories can be both liberating and healing (R. Atkinson, 1995; Charmaz, 1999; Epstein, 1995; Josselson & Lieblich, 1995; McLaughlin, 1996; Remen, 1996b). Both of us looked forward to our meetings in and out of the hospital. Our relationship fostered comfortable adjustments to accommodate the exigencies of Carol Ann's health status. Familiarity overcame concern about reactivity that might suggest the manipulating awareness or conspicuousness sometimes encountered in direct observation research (Gittelsohn, Shankar, West, Ram, & Gnywali, 1997; Kent & Foster, 1977). However, as respectful, caring, and open as we were with each other, there were definitive boundaries in our relationship.

As Carol Ann defined her need for a clinical counselor, a need which remained unmet until the end, that became a topic of consideration in our explicating the relationship we had. We acknowledged soon after her transplant surgery that I would not and should not be that clinical counselor, although many of our conversations might have been indistinguishable from those of people engaged in such a relationship. Carol Ann always introduced me to others as her dissertation chair and mentor, in later years adding "and friend" to that. She valued a separation of roles that acknowledged me as an academic researcher and herself either as participant or coresearcher, although she always qualified the latter with reminders of her own preparation in quantitative rather than qualitative approaches and methods. She consciously chose to maintain a view of me as teacher and herself as student and teaching assistant, presenting me, shortly after her discharge from the hospital (and less than a year following her graduation with a doctorate in nursing), with a needlepoint pillow that says "To teach is to touch a life forever."

It was not insignificant in our mutual caring and connecting that Carol Ann saw me as a healthy, European American, rural-rooted, married woman who was personally ungrounded in her (Carol Ann's) fervent Protestantism and, coming from a background in psychiatric–mental health and intercultural nursing (but perhaps more aligned with anthropology than nursing), clinically naive to the intricacies of intensive care nursing. She described herself, in contrast, as someone who had lived with a chronic illness from the age of 8; was African American, urban-oriented, and never married; had kept the Church of Christ central to her entire spiritual, social, and philosophical life; and, professionally, identified intensely with critical care nursing and loved every aspect of the biology and technology involved therein. Completely at home spewing laboratory values and physiological details, she would shake her head and chuckle at my ambivalence toward technology and thirst for glimpsing meaning in the larger picture. While our personal experiences with ethnicity and race had for years served as a meaningful bridge in our discourse, the religious–spiritual and nursing–technology differences in our disparate biographies both separated us and made us complementary. Although Carol Ann knew as well as I did that demands in my life realistically limited the energy available for a clinical facet in our relationship, it was her belief in emotional support as part of ethical clinical deliberation and sound healthcare, and her firm expectation that such support be provided *within* the healthcare organization—"and certainly any hospital fancy enough to have a transplant unit!" as she put it—that definitively and officially disqualified me from both the label and the overt task. Carol Ann, always one to comply with the letter of the law and abide by organizational structure, was quick to exceed minimum expectations but firmly resistant to accepting less. Her own needs and clinical situation aside, she expected (even demanded) that her healthcare be comprehensive, both in the hospital and after discharge, and to her that included, when needed, a psychosocial component that carried the same status and authority as her other care and treatment.

As is the case with nearly all qualitative inquiry, initiation of our interpretive work coincided with our earliest discussions around our decision to create a textual narrative of her experience with transplant. That interpretation continued until Carol Ann's death 4 years later, and even after that through input from Carol Ann's father and various readers of the evolving manuscript. Initially, turning to the phenomenon led to tracing etymological sources, searching idiomatic phrases, developing thick descriptions of experiences that were sometimes garbled in memory and muffled by physical weakness and emotional distress, and repeated telling of stories. Over time, those procedures allowed sharing of feelings and situations, exploring of possibilities not otherwise considered, and the detailing of unique and particular episodes while transcending the particularity of their storylines. My research task as conversational and interpretive partner was listening for the meaning of what was being said (Rubin & Rubin, 1995) and hearing the meanings, interpretations, and understandings that gave shape to Carol Ann's narrative of her experience. Moving back and forth between portions of the text and interpretations allowed cyclical confrontation and development of new interpretative questions (Benner & Wrubel, 1989; Denzin, 1997), as dialectic underlies interpretation and guides the process of inquiry, thus creating the hermeneutic circle. Akin to Heidegger's description of a perpetual oscillation of new perspectives being broadened, changed and specified, "the thing itself" emerges and guides interpretation (Heidegger, 1962).

Questioning, reflecting, focusing, and intuiting helped articulate and make explicit meanings embedded in Carol Ann's transplant experience and its sequelae, while the entire research transaction was strongly characterized by the openness, flexibility, and responsiveness of interpersonal reasoning (Noddings, 1991). We initiated our interpreting around van Manen's (1990) four essentials: lived space, lived body, lived time, and lived human relating. As interpreters, we consciously tried to balance acknowledging Carol Ann's needs with retaining a focus on our phenomenological and ethnographic objectives and avoiding digression into criticism or medical evaluation. Realizing a need to forestall journalistic exposé, as well as any insinuation of being antiscientific or antiresearch, we continually examined our own more revisionist goals and methods. The inquiry made us deeply mindful of what it means to be human when a person is situated as both professional and patient in the biomedical world of organ transplantation. As participants in the domain of professional healthcare, we had to guard against the text reflecting professional ideology or resembling our own versions of practice (Benner & Wrubel, 1989).

Initially, the object was, within our validating circle of inquiry, to transform Carol Ann's lived experience into a textual expression of its essence to produce, through interpretation, a reflective and meaningful, contextualized reliving of the phenomenon (Denzin, 1997; van Manen, 1990) of transplantation. However, my medical anthropological orientation and, as a teaching assistant, Carol Ann's familiarity with that stance led us to view our task as one of critique as well as interpretation. Just as nursing's history has evolved beyond its traditional emphasis on "women worthies" (Church, 1987), we—as nurses and women—liked to think that "the role of nursing in the health field is the epitome of women's role in American society" (Ashley, 1976, p. 125). But, as history is guided as much by moral inquiry as by science (Halttunen & Perry, 1999), self-knowledge of nursing's role, and the critique essential to knowing nurses and nursing within the context of healthcare, and to knowing healthcare within the contexts of biomedicine and of broader society, requires a critical (Joralemon & Fujinaga, 1996; Stevens, 1989), as well as an interpretive eye. For more than 3 years postdischarge and nearly 4 posttransplant, until Carol Ann's death in June 1999, we shared analyses and interpretations to explicate meanings in Carol Ann's everyday world of health professional as transplant patient, during which what really *mattered*—initially transplantation—evolved until it emerged as caring.

Although the uniqueness of the case study allows the significance and meaning of an experience to take precedence over objective fact (Ben-Ari, 1995), a case study cannot do justice to representing social process. The possibilities for interpretative stances are too many and varied. Stories are also notoriously individuated, while common understandings create their very worth (Bloom, 1996; Mishler, 1991). However, close scrutiny of an experience alleged to be patterned and shared by others modifies the risk of recounting and attending to what might be an isolated and iconoclastic experience. That is, it is often argued, if an experience is so unique and individualistic that no one else can relate to it, let alone is likely to experience it, the value of its description resides not in any potential to inform clinical practice but only in the academic, or perhaps even outside that as a curiosity for ingestion by lay readers. The design we settled on, or more accurately *into,* has some pronounced advantages regarding the authenticity and credibility of the research. Exercising personal history to understand and respond to each other reflects genuine caring behaviors that are congruent with particular attitudes, values, and beliefs, as well as provides purpose for focusing in particular directions (Hall, 1990). With unquestionable engagement with her own life experiences, Carol Ann as research participant became the center of the text creation and interpretive process, thus reinforcing the credibility of the procedure by enabling synthesis of her experience through contact and empathy (Patton, 1990; Swanson, 1991).

Since qualitative inquiry seeks to enter the world of the participant, it stands to reason that use of self as vessel or medium is important (Rew et al., 1993). On the other hand, acceptable intersubjective soundness is achievable through connection with cultural values and social norms inherent in the phenomenon serving as the focus of inquiry. As self-interpreting beings through and through, we *knew* the phenomenon we wished to *understand*. We were well versed in the context of meaning in which biomedicine, transplantation, treatment, and both care and caring occur. In Carol Ann's narrative, explicating interactions quickly brought caring (as distinct from either treatment or care) to the forefront by virtue of its presence, or at times, its relative absence or an anomalous presence. Making sense of care, caring, being-cared-for, and being-cared-about experiences, being open to insights into their shape, and getting to the basic nature and description of the phenomenon of caring during the transplant experience were essential to revealing the intricate unity of Carol Ann's lifeworld. It is experience that is co-constituting of person and his or her world (Heidegger, 1962). Yet the nature of the experience must be probed in its essential sections to grasp different aspects of the situation as those work in concert, albeit not necessarily in harmony. At the same time, it is the integration of the parts that tells the real story. Carol Ann's story is, for instance, neither the empathic professional's nor the medically impaired patient's. It is one of experience lived by a person with a life inclusive of, but extending beyond, both roles.

The Story

The first thing I remember was the phone call from the transplant coordinator. I panicked. I didn't know what to do first.

"I have a kidney and a pancreas for you."

"What do I do? What do I do?"

"We have a bed ready."

I drove myself to the hospital.

The healthcare providers in Carol Ann's story almost immediately become "*they*," the other—sometimes the other who cares, sometimes the other who brings pain and even danger—but always the *other*. The hospital became essentially surreal, the experience Kafkaesque in nature. There were multiple threats to the stability of bodily boundaries, the sense of self, feelings of humanity, and perceptions of reality. Carol-

Ann-as-patient and members of the transplant team often seemed to view situations in disparate ways. "You ask about 'they.' Am I who I thought I was? One of them? They control; when the only other option is doing nothing, they surely have the control."

Teaching hospitals have a lot of people around to poke and prod, to feel this and do that. There is not much allowance for dignity. Entire teams walk into my room, rip down my sheet, open up my wound, and leave me there for the nurse to redress the wound—all with the door wide open. . . . It is like treatment by gang warfare. They seem unaware and seem to think nothing of taking off the covers, probing through my wound site, baring everything I have. It is embarrassing to have 9 or 10 people even looking at me, let alone looking at my open wound. . . .

Docs don't really care much about pain and comfort. They are quick to say, "Oh, we can give you numbing medicine or an analgesic." They don't realize how invasive procedures can be, how inconvenient and distasteful, how just plain nasty, even without the pain.

Despite what Carol-Ann-as-health professional *knows*, her experience conveys that the medical and nursing professionals are preoccupied with the functioning of the transplanted organ. In short, only her kidney really *matters;* even her new pancreas is forgotten when it fails and is removed (although the surgeon later insisted it should not have been, "if only it had not been a weekend" and he had been alerted). Carol Ann felt that she, the woman the kidney resided in, and the experience of that *person,* became dissociated from the transplant. The entire process focused, she insisted, away from the patient and toward the transplanted body part in its new home among other biological body parts and subsystems.

When physicians use distancing as a coping strategy, they shift responsibility for the patient's emotional health, and its care, to the nurses (Moos, 1984). That does not mean that the nurses assume that responsibility or do so adequately to meet the patient's needs. In Carol Ann's experience, there was a powerful distancing in the nurses' superficial friendliness, strapped as it was by the sheer numbers of seriously ill patients they tried to manage in an environment strained in many ways. Despite occasional brusqueness, generally the nurses were pleasant, respectful, even cheerful . . . and still distant. There was a frankness that caring by nurses is illusory that bothered Carol Ann. It was too acute a reminder that carers do not get paid for caring or for being caring, but for providing efficient care. They are answerable to many people and have copious amounts of information at their fingertips. Numerous assumptions are made about what care patients need and want.

One source of disconnection is placement in hospital rooms. The nurses assume that privacy is more important than the emotional support I could get by being with others. The consequence is that I am isolated and left feeling alone. Having time to myself is often not what I need. That sense of being with, not being abandoned, is so vitally important here. I am always in private rooms except when I first came on the transplant unit. Then I was with another woman, another transplant patient, and we connected with each other through prayer and faith and our experience. But then the nursing staff disconnected us physically and emotionally in their effort to protect us.

In the hospital, Carol Ann lived with the fear that no one would come when she needed help. This sense of disconnection was reinforced by the staff when her physical isolation was justified by her development of MSRA (methicillin-resistant staphylococcus aureus [Jackson, Rickman, & Pugliese, 1999]). The nurses were no longer "totally at fault for isolating me; they were required to do so by infection control." As much as she resented the physicians' failure to provide some privacy, she *feared* nursing staff closing the door and leaving her alone. Despite understanding the risks and processes of infectious disease, Carol Ann lived with knowing that, with so much to do, *they* might or might not respond to her. Despite her own professional comfort with technology, its indulgence and the seemingly wanton time, knowledge, and other resources invested in sustaining that, appalled her. Carol Ann asked, "How can anyone *need* 15 CAT scans?" No one provided an adequate answer. Despite being subject to endless tests, there was little explanation of findings or follow-up on many of them.

I'm learning a lot about being truly sick. If I was ever truly sick before, I don't remember. I am 41, and I have had diabetes for 33 years, but I have not been *truly sick* until now. Being truly sick is to be so helpless that you can't lift your head up off the pillow and you don't care what they do to you. Mostly you are helpless. Hopelessly helplessly helpless. . . . If you are so sick that you cannot be vigilant, you are in real trouble because you are very vulnerable. Even when I am so sick, those times when I am really in and out of it—not completely aware of some things going on around me—I am still enough aware to know that I have to be my own best advocate. I know I have to try to maintain a handle on the treatment I am getting. On a couple of occasions, I probably saved my life when I've caught things on the brink of disaster. I remember being sick and having a blood glucose in the 20s or 30s and waking up and trying to convince the nurse that I needed some D[extrose]-50 or something to try to get my sugar up. It took an interminable amount of time for her to get a blood glucose, and by the time she got it, she really did not believe the number. I insisted that she go ahead and give me the D-50 and if I needed to chase it with insulin, fine, we would do so. Once, with a glucose of 37, they were ready to give me insulin. I said, "I think you need to rethink this." *I have to be the master of my own care,* in spite of the way I feel and how sick I am. I cannot be the nurse, yet I have to be.

I've become a pill counter, alert to and monitoring "strange" meds [medications] in my pill cups. This was okay when I was able to do this, when I was wide awake and not hallucinating, but who knows what could happen during my less lucid moments? *I wish I did not have to think about all this. . . .*

Being vigilant is about fearing that care will slip into carelessness and about the reserve-draining stress of keeping "half an eye open at all times." It is about craving for someone's *caring* about and for you, while knowing you have to rely on their *taking care of* you in physical and technological and even environmental terms. Being vigilant is about a maddening need for spiritual caring that no one seems to hear, a need for touching that no one seems to feel. Being vigilant is about waiting.

Waiting interminably. Of having nothing to do and to be about. The days are long but the nights are longer. Every 5 minutes can creep into hours, each moment, each hour hyper-extended. Waiting for care when what I really wanted was caring, *time* spent *caring.* Care is scheduled; caring is not. Caring is connecting, visiting, being there. It is what the secretaries or the techs do when they come into the room to chat before coming on or going off shift, or the wound care nurse who comes by to visit and check about my ileostomy. It is *being* together, not *doing* together. Granted, caring is not an easy job with all these complications of mine that divert attention. Some of the nurses genuinely try to make it better for me. They look up meds that are new to me in their drug books and tell me about them, although generally the nursing staff is happier when I direct my questions to medicine than to them. It must be just as hard for them sometimes to deal with the complications as it is for me. I have too much time to worry about these things, but it helps me mark the time.

You lose time in critical care. You lose days. You lose track because there are no cues. Sometimes I am able to see a clock so I know what time it is, but

I do not know whether it is night or day. Sometimes I can even see a window, depending on where I am: transplant, ICU [intensive care unit], or Intermediate ICU. But dusk and dawn look alike and winter days are short. You struggle to be oriented. Why aren't there calendars, time messages, some way of letting patients know who they are and where they are and when they are? *They* ask those questions all the time, but if you don't remember and have no clues, with all these drugs on board, it is astounding that anybody can keep the answers straight.

The irony is that way back in 1982, Carol Ann was quoted in an article explaining how to prevent ICU psychosis (Star, 1982). Time gaps are excruciating when one realizes what is happening but has no control over it. Although they did little to instill a sense of control in her life, one thing that marked Carol Ann's time was rounds, which included some 9 or 10 or more people, including auxiliary departments such as infectious disease, pharmacy, nutrition, and the renal or dialysis physicians, in addition to post graduate residents in their first, second, and third years. There was always at least one unit nurse and a transplant coordinator. The latter was a nurse practitioner who made sure the lab data were current and available to the surgeons. It took 3 hours to do rounds on this unit, for an average of 60 patients. The senior resident was in charge of multiple patient care areas and rotated through rounds on other transplant areas with different residents, while the three levels of post graduate residents stayed on the transplant unit, except for surgery.

The medical post grads, the new residents, can be like the Keystone Cops bumbling through: "Which way did he go, George? Which way did he go?" There are no real checks and balances. Physicians write orders and nurses carry them out. You presume they have been written and carried out correctly. But the system is complex and there are few checks on what staff really do. . . .

My everyday fear comes from having enough medical knowledge and experience *to know what is right and wrong for me.* I am probably the best person to know that, in spite of the doctors. I can't rely on my parents and others to be here in the middle of night, to know what questions to ask, to know how I feel, and to speak for me. And the staff and docs too seldom ask. It's very frightening. If *I* have this kind of knowledge about medical care, God bless the people who don't. I know physicians on call have all sorts of demands to which they must attend, and sometimes they make mistakes. But I don't want to be one of those medical mistakes. I don't want to be the "oops" that people talk about.

It seems that hospital teams aren't really teams. On one hand, they often don't have captains or the captains are not apparent; on the other hand, every "member" is too much an individual to know how to work together. Things get missed because each "team" member is doing his or her own thing. Despite the many players, there is no quarterback on any consistent basis. Or teams consult the captain only once a day, if that. Sometimes the chart is there, or at least they are carrying around someone's chart, but no one opens it and writes anything in it. They all seem to depend on the memories of residents, who have already been up the night before and it's now 4 PM. . . . Nurses won't do anything unless the order is written down, and it is the physician's responsibility to write the order in the chart. Communication is not their strength. They think and say they were all working together, but it is like parallel play. Superficial. Technical togetherness, all in the same place but disconnected.

There were nurse managers on the transplant unit. They have managerial expertise but not necessarily clinical expertise, which was a bone of contention among the staff RNs [registered nurses]. The unit RNs were responsible for juggling patients according to acuity level. They determined who went to the subacute side of the unit. However, the transplant coordinators, nurse practitioners [NPs] with prescription-writing privileges, came from outside the hospital. They were part of the surgical team in an office *near* the hospital, but they were not part of the nurses providing care on the transplant unit. The NPs are the initial transplant contact and dealt with preliminary lab data and work-ups, "stress tests and all that to facilitate admission." Although presumably the most educated and expert nurses about transplant, on the unit they could merely make suggestions. There was also little apparent coordination between the transplant coordinating NPs and the transplant RNs who took over on the unit. The latter were diverse, some trained in critical care and transplant, but others from the pool or "travelers." They recovered patients who did not need post-surgery ICU. "But I always seem to go to ICU after surgery . . ."

The nurses did nothing without a written order. The medical residents stayed off the floor, being in surgery early in the day. So rounds did not occur until late afternoon. Then the residents' notes might or might not be recorded in the chart in time to be acted on that day. There were chart rituals but no record at the bedside for medications. There was an on-call transplant surgeon, a task that switched on a weekly basis. The surgeon addressed the post graduate interns; the chart was present for consulting. But the residents were more likely to make notes

on their 3-by-5 cards than in the chart. One wonders who is intended
to benefit from such rituals. Is it the physician in quest of a firmer knowledge for future practice (Warner, 1997), or the patient living with an
inconveniently—even inconsiderately—unpredictable present and perhaps too terrified to envision a future?

Carol Ann believed that the transplant coordinators and many other
team members related to her situation differently than they would if she
were not a health professional. That created another level of problems.
Relating to a shared professional perspective did not facilitate understanding personal experience; indeed, it may help avoid that connection.
Carol Ann was aware of a sense of urgency stemming from depression
and futility. She felt guilty over what her parents were going through
and angry that no one listened to her most of the time in the hospital—
even when she called out explicitly for emotional support. She believed
her surgeon actually treated her preferentially, yet direct requests for
a supportive counseling consult, specifically for "someone to talk to
about all this," resulted in his telling "me to just let out a scream and
it will all be okay. If only it were so easy!" So treatment meant seemingly
unlimited laboratory tests and medical trial and error, but no counseling
consult. "It cuts away at me and I am pulled into a scenario that will
not allow me to be who I am. I can't deal only with the physical without
the emotional." Yet Carol Ann also found pleasure in the trusting and
somewhat collegial relationship she developed over time with the surgeon. Although it failed to provide the type and level of care she needed
and may have indicated frank relief on his part that accusation and litigation were not looming on the horizon, she felt it also provided her some
protection. She learned it was futile to express her emotions and sus-
pected that only "nice neat patient patients" are cared about, as well as
cared for. But she resented the avoidance of responsibility by members
of several disciplines that resulted in medical and nursing mistakes.

Sometimes they wanted to know something that had no effect on the plan of
action, and I would refuse. They would be furious. One cannot help but wonder
whether they would stop treating you if you made too big a stink.

The patient and professional in me merged. To have dressing changes done
diligently, I often have to insist. Sometimes I am pushed by the medical staff,
other times they sit back to see what happens.

Transplantation did not diminish Carol Ann's awareness of being a
member of society in a particular time and place. She shared the cultural

orientations of being American and African American, as well as the confused social status and role of both health professional and patient. Every aspect of her history and biography fed into the decisions she made and her experience with illness. As such, she could not be viewed in an extracted, isolated set of circumstances. Carol Ann commented often about how many patients with end stage renal disease are persons of color and how few there were on the transplant unit (Johnson, Wicks, Milstead, Hartwig, & Hathaway, 1998). Yet, throughout the prolonged hospitalization, Carol Ann was never asked her race or ethnicity. An African American woman in the admissions office indicated on one admission form that Carol Ann was "black," while someone else on the transplant unit described her in the chart as "white." The latter label persisted, appearing months later in the discharge record.

The environment seems to purposely disconnect. Caring *could* preserve my personal and my cultural expressions of illness. Caring people *could* support my family during all these painful events. Some nurses and physicians are uncertain of my background, my race and culture. They did not seem to know to whom or where I belong—and, oddly, they did not know to ask or how to ask. Once it was written down, the first line of every description bore a mistaken assumption: "41-year-old white woman." It does not matter medically except for those few diseases that tend to be racially patterned, but *it matters to me.* They should not mislabel if they are going to label. They obviously decided what race they thought I was or they wanted me to be; they surely did not ask. Then they went about giving care from a European American perspective. The failure to find out and preserve my identity seems disrespectful to me; it is a failure of care to be so insensitive.

It is as if, with the essentials of care dutifully rendered in the here and now, the patient's past and future become irrelevant. To various extents, the *person*-object of care, being little more than a surrogate for (or a shell containing) *a patient,* becomes invisible (K. Davis, 1993)—so invisible that such a patient-casing might be overlooked or misplaced. At times, recognition and acknowledgment of Carol Ann's very existence seemed to extend beyond the present-oriented call of duty. Here I interject a visitor's perspective.

I went to see Carol Ann on the transplant unit after work one day, only to discover her missing. None of the staff knew where she was. She was on and off this unit for *months*—more on than off—and she was there last evening, and *tonight no one questioned where she's gone.*

She was not present to be cared for, that much was known. "There was no mention of her in report." Accountability beyond that apparently exceeded realistic expectations. Yet Carol Ann had been so ill during the past several days that it would not have surprised me to be told she had died, passed on, expired. But on the transplant floor, I was welcomed as any other familiar visitor might be after having been there scores of times. No one seemed to realize that *I did not go to visit the transplant unit,* but to visit Carol Ann, a person I'd only yesterday seen in the care of the staff of that unit. I found myself having trouble asking, "Did she die?" and wondered why they did not tell me. They would know, should know, if she died, *wouldn't they?* Doubts haunted my conviction, little doubting side effects of the untrusting, confusing gaps spawned by so many levels of intimacy juxtaposed with so much confusion and superficial relating. I told myself to trust the mechanics, the business of the place—that any retail business worth its salt would know how many transactions occurred today, or what goods were transferred to other departments. I tried to convince myself that it was irrational to expect the staff to know what had become of one of the dozen or so people for whom they provided total care last night on the more acute side of the transplant unit.

With her record gone from the unit, there was no evidence that Carol Ann had ever been there. The ward clerk was at dinner, and the staff, many of them unfamiliar to me despite my nearly nightly visits, was busy. I knew it was ridiculous, but I was afraid to go to the lobby's patient information desk for fear they might blunder into denying that she ever was here. I chided myself for too many mysteries listened to on my long commutes. I waited in the hall until the ward clerk returned and I could press her to search the patient record on my behalf. Sure enough, Carol Ann had again been transferred to an ICU, this time a different one of the half dozen scattered about the medical center. In a facility in which technology can image any organ and physiology has few secrets, it took 50 minutes to determine where an entire specific person, a person who when last seen did not have the capacity to transport herself anywhere, had been *put.*

Over time, her social identity carelessly propelled into mechanistic and bureaucratic limbo, Carol Ann struggled to deal with a greatly altered self. Physically, she maintained an adequate body weight, but medications tended to lump it in the abdominal area and face, while her limbs thinned. Living with clothing that hung in places no matter how accurate its size, Carol Ann described her appearance as akin to "a prisoner of war with kwashiorkor." The pressure to eat was not helped by taking large quantities of medications and contending with subsequent severe gastrointestinal upsets.

My body image has really gone berserk. I look at myself in the mirror and see stigmata, a scar from my breasts to my pubis and another one where the ileostomy was. Puncture marks all over my body. My midline incision is coming together finally, but my navel is downright funky.

With Carol Ann finally discharged, the nurse practitioner transplant coordinators took over. Problems were directed to them through phone paging. They triaged to the emergency rooms, office, clinics, consults, and home care. The transplant coordinators became Carol Ann's single consistent and reliable connection with nurses, yet they are not RNs employed by the medical center for the transplant unit but functioned *outside the hospital* and, in response to the surgical team's transplant coordinators' mandate to check daily the laboratory results of *all* transplant team patients, they notified those patients with abnormal results. Despite this one area in which Carol Ann could rely on nurses to make contact, it was long in being revealed, for it had to wait for discharge and was strictly limited.

Carol Ann knew that all transplant nurses' roles included patient support and counseling. She heard them describe emotional, psychological, and social aspects of their roles. All were very friendly, yet they too failed to connect on a level she needed because the empathic communication she longed for was compromised by an inability to allow time for caring. The resources were simply not there: "They don't have the time or the energy." The failure to connect with her directly dominated her experience with the transplant coordinating NPs, as it did with the unit nurses. "But they follow-up well on lab data, even when they otherwise are not present, and their efforts, based as they are on unfocused or too narrowly focused assessments, sometimes go awry." Although Carol Ann said she was "past knee-jerking to crises," several times she was upset severely by the transplant NPs' urgent messages, left on Carol Ann's phonemail system, indicating abnormal values in her lab work that threatened "dire consequences." One message, delivered with urgency but mechanically on the day after Christmas required a hurried return to the hospital only to be kept waiting there for more than a day before anything was done. "They clearly are more invested in those numbers than they are in me or my response to their frantic messages. They want me to get my body in there. They don't much care if I'm psychologically traumatized in the process."

Not taking the time that Carol Ann associated with caring, "being there," was a recurrent theme. It often made the difference between feeling cared for and cared about. However, another level of brusque efficiency fostered even greater distancing, particularly when Carol Ann and the medical personnel did not share common treatment goals.

It's like it is with doctors who give pat answers so that they don't feel blamed for the pain they cause. But it becomes routine, those answers. . . . People are stressed out trying to do too much with too many very sick patients. Judgment is sacrificed to get the tasks accomplished; the need for control kicks in.

Reflecting deep fears after her six major surgeries, Carol Ann had ominous dreams of being rehospitalized. The surgeries melted into an indistinct single experience, and many issues remained unresolved. She tried not to think about them, yet was aware of a need to talk about the very things she least liked dwelling on. Despite her expertise and experience in critical care nursing and a doctorate focused on nursing ethics, after her prolonged surgical experience she regarded the ideal life as one she imagined a concierge to have, "someone who arranges people's lives for them on vacation, or maybe a caterer"—a diabetic caterer who understands dietary boundaries while making the most of living creatively within them. But her energy level precluded developing those positive dreams. A year and a half posttransplant, knowing the rate at which she moved, Carol Ann, an accomplished cook, got up at six in the morning to begin preparations for the lunch we shared at noon. She shopped frequently in small amounts, since even brief standing resulted in uncomfortable edema in her legs. Two and a half years posttransplant, she was still taking 35 pills a day, and cellulitis and stress fractures were taking new tolls. Three years posttransplant, who she was remained in painful transition. Not being able to accept herself as disabled, Carol Ann resisted using a wheelchair shopping cart. Only when desperation outweighed reluctance did she request a handicapped sticker for parking. An insidious awareness of the chronicity of her diminished health status lingered and thrived.

Sometime after my third surgery, I said to my father, "Take the kidney out. I don't want the responsibility." I realized for the first time how much time and effort it will take just to take care of me on a daily basis. I can't do it and have a full-time job. I feared I would not be able to handle all of the responsibility. I don't want people to think that transplants aren't a good thing, but you've really got to have your head together—and someone to help it stay that way.

Carol Ann's life continued to be shaped by the transplant experience. She wondered at and worried about the ramifications. Whereas previously she monitored the acuity of her diabetes and failing renal situation, health issues later were grounded as much in the transplant as in the diabetes. Each had its own set of criteria for immediacy and onset of problems. No longer able to trust her body to respond in predictable ways, Carol Ann came to value plans—any plan, any day—because a plan meant advanced warning while surprises foretold disappointment, delay, missed meals, and bad news. Despite years of effectively managing her diabetes, she was shocked and mortified to experience a severe insulin reaction during a public meeting in which she had a part. After developing kidney disease and the subsequent transplant, sensations warning of a plummeting blood glucose level took longer to manifest themselves. Without familiar cues, even a much experienced, highly knowledgeable, long-term diabetic was left having to be increasingly cautious and feeling decreasingly prepared and confident. Control was limited, and there were new fears of doing something embarrassing or dangerous in the kaleidoscope of activities outside her control. With her "normal-for-me diabetic life" replaced by something ominously unruly, so much was out of control that nearly any predictability was worthy of preservation.

Dialysis was a continuation of my diabetes, an extension of that. Dialysis made me look at time differently, but other things were not so different. But this [transplant] experience has changed my outlook. Taking care of myself is a full-time job. How I look at my recovery is changing; patience is hard to master, but at least now crises come one at a time, not in multiples—at least usually. It is a progression of things and not all at once. My parents are encouraging me to rely on other people; I am getting pushed out of the nest again. I have to take on more of the responsibilities, the logistics of blood draws and appointments, the finances, the calls from doctors' offices when paperwork goes astray. I hope that eventually I can streamline this taking care of myself. I went to visit friends this weekend as a trial run. It increased my confidence in both my ability and that of my friends to be able to help. The goal is to be able to take care of myself and have a full-time job. It gets frustrating. I can't imagine doing it.

Before this experience, everything was centered around work and my job. Who I was, was what I did. The Protestant work ethic, working at being. My old meaning meant being a productive member of society, contributing to professional nursing through education. Now it means taking care of myself to be able to return to being a productive member of society. And it means fearing that may never happen. I am different, more self-centered. . . . I set little goals, such as walking into the DMV [Department of Motor Vehicles] without a cane to renew my driver's license. It is a test of patience. Anytime I don't take things slowly and patiently enough, I land on the floor.

I know there is no shame in taking time to heal, despite the pressure to cost less. I am more sensitive to people with problems than I ever was before, but I am jealous of those who heal readily and can be back to being who they are. Healing needs sensitivity; it does not happen by lab numbers alone. The challenge is to question without complaining. To get myself together for whatever is next. To move on. It takes more to pull yourself together for each step than the docs ever imagine. People really don't want normal reactions to what happens in healthcare. They want heroics.

Carol Ann pointed out that out-patient status allowed the luxury of reflecting on the meaning of her experience with less distraction by the experience itself. "I'm more introspective in my thinking, less focused on survival than when I was so vulnerable."

Once I was discharged, I got better—when I was treated less aggressively. After I told them that I could not financially afford being hospitalized so much, they seem to have become less concerned about the numbers, and they gave me a little more leeway. But still, when I tell them I feel good and they tell me I look good, whoosh!—they readmit me because of the numbers. Sometimes I think I can survive this if they would leave me alone to heal. When they discontinue a medication, often the problem goes away. Now I have a list. One doc says, "Don't let anyone give you this"; another says, "Never let anyone put you on that." I do worry about problems with the anti-rejection drugs versus the immunosuppressant balance. But *they* always want to treat the numbers; rarely, very rarely am I asked *how I really feel*. So we wait for new numbers. The threat of being called into the hospital at a moment's notice controls my life. My level of wellness or illness determines my response to everything. I take all *their* news with a grain of salt because they don't know what is going on with me, and they don't know any more than I do what will happen, but it still controls my life. I am their experiment. I have to play wait and see—see the numbers, see what happens when they treat the numbers, which is what they always treat. *It's what they really care about.*

Interpreting, or What the Biocultural Body Tells

Transplantation, although increasingly common, carries with it mind-boggling implications and questions around embodiment and the boundaries of personhood. Whether transcending or simply breaking social expectations, transplantation is no simple gift, for gift-exchange transactions exact reciprocity that society denies in organ replacement where the recipient is seldom heard from (Ohnuki-Tierney, 1994). Renal transplantation is replete with threats of rejection, complex medical regimes, and demands for on-going medical supervision, yet its regalia of analytical and technical literature encompasses virtually no chronicle of patient responses to transplantation and to postsurgical sequelae (Fallon, Gould, & Wainwright, 1997).

Meanwhile, the technology of transplantation enacts myriad cultural transgressions, calling into question basic understandings of what is human and non-human, rational and emotional, life and death, self and other, and natural and unnatural (Kleinman, 1995). Given this sea of ambiguity, of being neither here nor there, one wonders at the missing voices of those who have endured the transformation of transplant and are living with other peoples' organs in them. Surely these are more than replacements for nonfunctioning parts, and Gadamer (1996) is correct about the "limitations of objectification." Human experience, in its manifest variety, cannot be solidified into an assemblage of theorems (Adorno, 1973; Jackson, 1996) or technical reasoning (Beverley, 2000) to be presented as scientific artwork. Realization that experiences and meanings can flow from unlikely places, and that little is absolute, sacred, permanent or truly sealed off in solitary existence, has left earlier commitments to objectivism in doleful doubt (Denzin & Lincoln, 2000).

Exploring living with the knowledge of being in a life-threatening situation is not a new idea (Groopman, 1997; Reed, 1991; Running, 1996; Scott-Maxwell, 1968). Such stories, and the questions they prompt, resonate with curious trajectories toward ennoblement and defeat, or sometimes both, at the hand of fate in the form of illness (Groopman, 1997). But *what* are those stories? *Where* are the stories of transplant and all of its challenges and complexities? "Clinical tales" tend to be minimized for their verbosity, avoided as undisciplined, or even treated with contempt by more objective aspects of scientific medicine (Sacks, 1985). Yet those narratives afford fuller accounts of patients' experiences than are reflected in statistics, lab reports, X-rays, and other nonnarrative fundamentals (Frank, 1995; Morris, 1998). Carol Ann's story is such a narrative, reaching as it does into deep and shadowy regions of healthcare that only lived experience can reveal.

Being Lost in the Crowded Mechanics of Care

Historically unprecedented dilemmas arise almost too quickly to be recognized, let alone resolved, in postmodern medicine. A few decades ago, heroic physicians and researchers fought to rescue patients and the world from disease. Today's medical practice is far more confusing and complicated with "painful moments of breakdown and failure" (Morris, 1998, p. 278). Society contends, as well as it can, with massive, disruptive, often abstract social change as medicine continues its migration from its sacred origins to regular membership in the industrial park (Davis-Floyd & St. John, 1998; Stein, 1995).

Critical illness, leaving no aspect of a patient's life untouched (Frank, 1991), brings a demanding paradoxical and clamorous duplicity into living (Sacks, 1995). While serious illness seriously complicates life, the therapeutic objectives in Western society have traditionally emphasized simplification, a "doing *with* the body only part of what needs to be done *for* the person" (Frank, 1991, p. 8). The alternative to compartmentalized medical specialization is an acknowledgment that actual *competence* in medicine is increasingly ambiguous (M.-J. D. Good, 1998). Anxiety over not knowing what to do reigns. Situations occur and questions are asked that would have been unthinkable in the past. Carol Ann's "Which way did he go, George? Which way did he go?" parodies the disorganization inherent in the very attempt to organize competent, complex intervention.

One thing that matters is the common thread among myriad views of biomedicine: its role in social control (Kleinman, 1995), "in shaping the regulation of human action, the deportment of human bodies and the construction of subjectivity" (Lupton, 1994, p. 19). Carol Ann, who lived with her body for more than four decades and with diabetes for more than three, and who managed both well enough to be a successful practicing clinician and to earn a Ph.D., was very rarely asked her opin-

ion of her own situation and even more rarely listened to or heard. Carol
Ann said:

Choices are a real issue in the hospital. I've had so many invasive procedures
that I've signed a lot of consent forms, but rarely did I have real choices. Not
all treatment options leave viable choices. The choices that are sometimes given
to me are not choices at all. They seem to present only one way of resolving
an issue. We talk about alternative treatments but often there are none; you
either get what they plan to do or you don't, the latter being labeled "conserva-
tive treatment." Usually the team has discussed a plan of action that they fully
intend to carry out; the effort then goes into bringing you along into their predetermined program. Choices are not really choices, just as the choice between
living and dying is not really a choice for me. I want to live. Not giving up is
part of me. . . . It is not an option. I can't really let go, although sometimes I
cannot hang on as tightly as I want to.

Values are identifiable in any everyday life experiences and consum-
erism's "more is better" orientation caricatures the sheer immensity of
medical meccas with their polish and science masking a bewildering
combining of the ordinary with the macabre. The popular view of disease as a culmination of sinister life struggles and social text evokes an
uneasy response to a surgical view of a body as mechanically broken but
fixable (Sontag, 1978; Stein, 1990). *"Thank goodness, and thanks to us,"*
Carol Ann quipped about medical godliness, while the pervasive chore
of getting functional again weighed heavily. Fixing became the object,
the basis for curing (albeit neither caring nor healing). However, hospitals, for all their mechanics, are not garages. "Fixing is a form of judgment" (Remen, 1996a, p. 24) that requires distance and disconnection.
Physicians freely and routinely overtreat, as far as funding allows, in
practicing "defensive medicine" (Schwartz, 1998).

Despite concern about nurses' accountability for professional practice (Cohen, Hausner, & Johnson, 1994), nursing and nurses, like
stretched rubber bands, are constantly taking on more tasks and responsibilities. The challenge to accomplish anything is greater but that to
accomplish *everything* is hypnotic, and the costs are insidious (Zalumas,
1995). Feeling that they and what they do is important hazards a re-
birthing of the old tension between altruism and autonomy, that is, trying to serve without being subservient (Rafael, 1996; Reverby, 1987b).
There is little space for connecting and touching and less for acknowl-

edging the real and incessant threat of death (Hauerwas, 1979; Moos, 1984). The serious possibilities of being "the 'oops' that people talk about" are more likely to be couched in legal than personal terms.

Intensifying the already strained carer's role, critical care involves a constancy of need and care of complicated patients in specialized, rapidly changing and complex environments, while nursing remains in the shadow on the sidelines where the moral, social, and ethical dimensions of decision making are seldom clear (Zalumas, 1995), yet interactions with patients are intimate and powerful human experiences of care (Lawler, 1993). There simply is not time for capturing the essence of human experience or the energy for holding it. So, etched in Kafkaesque reality, the signs of society's restructuring toward technical ways around an economic nucleus leave stressed carers lacking the support necessary to overcome depleted emotional reserves (Drew, 1986). The resulting insensitivity to patient responses is neither reassuring nor gratifying, but it can be explained away, rationalized through views of suffering that, while varying widely with circumstances, revolve around a dialectic between being over-involved and interfering with professional functioning, on one hand, and professional distance on the other (Baillie, 1996; Cohen et al., 1994; Kahn & Steeves, 1986; Steeves, Kahn, & Benoliel, 1990).

In everyday critical care reality, personal space is sacrificed willingly and without critique to the machines that make the seemingly impossible possible, that do what the sick body cannot, will not, or may not do. Noise levels mount despite *knowing* that sick people are less tolerant of noise than healthy people. Sensory overload contributes to feelings of helplessness, hopelessness, emotional lability, headaches, hallucinations, and sleep disturbances of myriad forms (Halm & Alpen, 1993). Carol Ann notes, however, that "At night there are fewer things to do and people to see, but docs are notorious for ordering tests at two in the morning." A narrow balance between sensory overload and sensory deprivation leaves one struggling to *be* in an environment where person-as-patient may seem little more than a means to an end.

Unlike healers of other traditions, practitioners of biomedicine experience a therapeutic environment in which moral goals of healing have been in large part replaced by technical and bureaucratic objectives (Davis-Floyd & St. John, 1998) that routinize the "quality" of care (Kleinman, 1995, p. 35). It is, meanwhile, the easiest way out. Transplant

technology, replete with questions as it is, would seem almost free of
the risk of being assumed a "value free endeavor" (Lock, 1997, p. 210).
Yet human history is one of choosing concealment, misunderstanding,
and even alienation. With culture reflecting the "collective experience
of everyday routines and rhythms of social life" (Kleinman, 1995, p. 54),
there is cultural continuity in the persistent valuing of impersonal (often
interpreted in common usage as synonymous with "professional") and
scientific principles of management in healthcare (Stein, 1995). A person who gets care but cries for caring denotes a patient who is either
a pawn or has been more or less forgotten in the fray. In Carol Ann's
case, not only did she lose her sense of situatedness, but she was at
times seemingly *lost*, no longer merely reduced to being numbered but
altogether misplaced, *transplanted* without a destination and a place to
be, as into the wrong greenhouse. Neither here nor there. Fear of being
lost extended to death. That fear of "nursing staff closing the door and
leaving" her alone was so poignant that it at times recollected Philippe
Ariès's (1977/1981) analysis of premedieval deaths characterized by terror. Whose person and voice was that Carol Ann envisioned closing the
door? Today's narratives, like Carol Ann's, speak to new old fears: being
trapped in liminal states where "living and dying obscenely commingle:
a contemporary version of the live burial" (Morris, 1998, p. 274).

That there is a need for attention to artful caring in these fragmen-
tary, consumer-oriented, power-focused, information- and technology-
ridden times of postmodern healthcare is an inevitable (N. Fox, 1993)
albeit unintentional situation (Lister, 1997). Pressure to increase patient
flow and productivity that is measured in narrowly defined biomedical
outcomes strongly parallels the time and motion studies inflicted on U.S.
industrial workers nearly a century ago (Stein, 1995; Taylor, 1911). That
Carol-Ann-as-patient and the transplant team often seem to view the
same situation in greatly disparate ways, and that really it is only her
new kidney that matters, is hardly surprising in the mass production of
outcomes-measured functions of care. Carol Ann is an artifact required
to keep the kidney going without resorting to yet more Kafkaesque inge-
nuity. It worked, urine was produced. *"Carol Ann is peeing!"* giggled
Carol Ann. "I remember being so excited that, as soon as I came out
of anesthesia, I called attention to my *full foley* to anyone who was
around!" It seemed as if that satisfied the medical folks; what more,
after all, can be asked of a kidney than that it produce urine? It is as if

such a successfully functioning kidney as this masterful replacement should have nothing to do with emotional responses. With all due respect to the dichotomy or unity of mind and body, emotions belong on another unit.

Science makes it easy for Carol Ann's physicians, functioning as they do in the culture of biomedicine, to *not* see or hear her needs for a counseling consult. Technically, arranging for the support of a social worker or counselor seems far simpler than transplant surgery, but the reason for and the reasonableness of the request eludes the mind set on science alone. The issue is a broader one, however, than a single surgeon repeatedly denying needed and requested support. If said physician reads primarily medical literature, he may not be aware of the research indicating such a need. Many of the studies assessing posttransplant quality of life have indicated serious problems in that area, yet medical journals have continued to publish reports that almost unanimously conclude that transplant recipients enjoy a high quality of life (Fallon et al., 1997; Joralemon & Fujinaga, 1996). Medical specialization, like any funneled attentiveness, sacrifices breadth for depth in the speed-up of complexity. But in a world focused on medical determination of *what is wrong with* somebody, Carol Ann talked about knowing "what is right or wrong *for me*," and she was not heard.

Carol Ann's story crystallizes a large-scale cultural conflict within which care becomes an autonomous, nearly concrete thing. Despite "a widening gap between what is medically possible and what is medically customary" (Schwartz, 1998, p. 63), intensive and critical care now comprise the usual standard of care in the U.S.A., while specialized techniques and technical imperatives can squeeze the caring out of nursing (Moorhouse, Geissler, & Doenges, 1987; Tisdale, 1986). Caring, and the time it takes for *being with* someone, is lost to the same inattention typically afforded the housecleaning brigade (Messing, 1998), for "*what* knowledge is attended to tends to be subordinate to *whose* knowledge" (Stein, 1995, p. 131). Social status and role are no less issues in health-care today than they have been in the past.

Historically, members of low-status disciplines have endured status anxiety analogous to that characteristic of marginal ethnic and racial groups in the U.S.A. (Stein, 1995). Nurses are accused of being too uncritical, or too blithely accepting, of the values of science and cultural materialism and of being so ready to accept overwhelming technical responsibilities that humanistic practice may be left to languor. In any event, accomplishing tasks seems so deeply ingrained in nurses, and in American women's roles, that it continually drowns out nurses' assertions of rights to determine their own activities (Broom, 1991; Corea, 1985; K. Davis, 1993; Fagin, 1975; Fisher, 1986; Fisher, 1995; Martin, 1987; Reverby, 1987a, b; Tomlinson, 1999).

What is salient, what *matters*, is oriented to the situation (Benner & Wrubel, 1989). Carol Ann's experience and her yearning for caring can be interpreted with Hanneman's (1996) description of patterns of expert practice as characterized by a minimal preoccupation with tasks and a strong emphasis on presence within a patient situation. Integral to this sense of "being there" is a familiarity with and sensitivity to a patient's responses with focused assessments, awareness of the interrelatedness and possibilities of situations, and decisive action guided by vigorous attention to patient outcomes (Hanneman, 1996). The nurse and the patient situation are, in other words, connected in a manner that allows empathy or an understanding of what the other person is *experiencing* (Baillie, 1996) or *suffering with* (Lane, 1987). In that situation, tasks become secondary to knowing; they are slighted so that thoughtful acting and interacting can reveal the lived meanings of a specific human experience (Sandelowski, 1997). As embodied knowing encompasses skillful comportment and perceptual and emotional responses (Benner & Wrubel, 1989), it is the nature of the human experience that becomes pre-eminent. Nonexpert practice, in contrast, involves less connection with (or even absence from) the patient situation, assessment that leaves patient responses in the background, and restrained action guided by a strong orientation to tasks and skills (Hanneman, 1996).

Carol Ann described, both as an in-patient and out-patient, an emphasis on physiological measures that repeatedly neglected, or obviated, her actual experience with a given situation. Whether or not the carers involved would agree with Carol Ann's take, the fact remains that she was very rarely consulted about *her* emotional and psychological responses to what was happening. From Carol Ann's perspective, the interweaving of inner experience and outer social reality left her suffering, estranged from the discourse of healthcare. The subsequent experience of a lack of connecting and caring on the part of those officially providing care is almost ironic in the world where embodied social practices, postures, and gestures should be fostering skillful perception and communication. But Carol Ann waited longingly and often in vain for interactions revealing the responses she expected in situations meaningful to her.

While caring may be what is sought from nurses and physicians, it is not the priority that is taught and learned as they are socialized to professional identities and grasp the intricacies of their work where the cultural values are embedded in the organization of time and the intensified urgency of innumerable deadlines fostering treatment of cases rather than people (Lupton, 1994).

One of the overarching "subjects" taught in the medical, internship, and residency curriculum is time. Indeed, a large part of the metacurriculum is *the experience of time.* In the typical seven-year (or more) process of medical training, students, interns, and residents are preoccupied with time. There is never enough time to do all one wants, is asked, and feels responsible to do. Throughout medical education, students, interns, and residents reckon time via a "countdown" of how long they have to go before some end is reached. Time is marked in short-term intervals, from one hurdle to the next. (Stein, 1990, p. 186)

There is no question that knowledge and technology are expected and demanded too. But temporality for Carol-Ann-as-patient, altered as it was with illness and etching timeless paths of loneliness, dictated meanings differently than might have been the case for Carol-Ann-as-professional in other circumstances. So when care went on autopilot and turned into cookie-cutter replications, even proscribed clinical paths were lost in cold and plasticized *applications and procedures* that Carol Ann responded to as hegemonic one-way acts upon her.

Doing Violence, Seeking Peace

Zalumas (1995, pp. 91–92) recites Margaret Mead's 1956 address to a national nursing conference, which, nearly a half century later, sounds far more bucolic than today's frenzied world, yet speaks to the protection, both somatic and psychic, that Carol Ann longs for:

I have tried to identify this thing that everybody who is a nurse does, and how the service you give to our society could be phrased. It seems to me that you protect the vulnerable, that you protect all those who are or could be in danger, in any kind of danger—from illness, from strain, from shock, from fatigue, from sorrow, from grief; that every spot in this society where there are those who are in danger and who need continuous concern, this is the place where you might function.

It is widely held today that healthcare is increasingly a matter of individual responsibility, the responsible adult being somehow capable and accountable for what happens, for his or her own health and well-being (Lowenberg, 1992), albeit that being sometimes beyond reasonable expectations. Carol Ann lamented, "I have to be the master of my own care, in spite of the way I feel and how sick I am. I cannot be the nurse, yet I have to be." The line between respecting patient determination and coercion is a narrow one requiring constant renegotiation with changing circumstances.

Victimization in care takes many forms. It can occur as the unintended consequence of thinking one is doing good while actually wreaking destruction, as can easily happen when mechanically providing personless, procedure-centered care and treatment. It can also occur when the patient's situation is used as leverage to promote a medical agenda over self-determination. Carol Ann said repeatedly that "Usually the team has discussed a plan of action that they fully intend to carry out; the effort then goes into bringing you along into their predetermined program." The line between productive and coercive power relations (Lupton, 1994) thins when recitations on self-care and personal responsibility give way.

The new ideology of choosing and its shifting attributions, although coming from a phenomenological and existential stance, retains an unresolved ambiguity. The physician is less responsible and less able to absolve patients from blame, while the sick are left more alone to survive their feelings of guilt or moral failure for becoming ill or for not healing, along with guilt for lifestyle lapses, and every imaginable stigma of their disability (Lowenberg, 1992). Even those with the knowledge to make informed choices about treatment may experience the available excesses of information as a moral burden (Lynn & Teno, 1993; Marshall, 1992). Understanding is linked to egalitarian relationships and mutuality in interaction that insinuate impracticality, if not impossibility, in medically dominated arenas.

Society continues to moralize experience, hence the portrayal in popular culture of physicians as thoroughly invested in moral dilemmas of patients and communities, while real life biotechnical values claim independence from such "parochial passions" (Kleinman, 1995, p. 35). The dialectic lurking in the precarious negotiation between consequences of sickness and its treatment is susceptible to dissolution. Like paradigmatic slashes, *doing to* and *doing for* poise to intersect *doing with*, rendering with a single stroke caring into naked care while remnants of stigmatizing illness and attributions of blame refuse to give up the old moral components of being sick (Siegler & Osgood, 1973). On the present surface, personal knowledge is disparaged and ignored, irreverently sacrificed to the preeminence of traditional biomedically dominated models of care and treatment.

Carol Ann, an intelligent, credentialed healthcare professional found her efforts at exercising power within contemporary biomedicine depressing and futile. No one with authority listened to her anger or absolved her of guilt over her role, imagined though it may have been, or of what she also imagined her parents were going through. There was no convincing reassurance from her healthcare providers that it was all right to relax and heal, to let down one's guard and concentrate on healing her wound rather than protecting it. Protective and paternal care providing involves efforts to defend against problems associated with *receiving* care and is viewed both as heroic and as a vital staving off of undesired potential consequences of care, such as acknowledged loss of control (Russell, Bunting, & Gregory, 1997). So while the patient's self-determination is increasingly socially and legally acknowledged on one hand, the bureaucratic and hierarchical dynamics perpetuate biomedicine's historical assumption of social control on the other.

Some people find in personal trauma an impetus for self-renewal (Jaffe, 1985). Such transformation follows wounding that occurs when one is wrenched out of taken-for-granted ordinary life and thrust into a nightmare in which the emotional defenses and sense of self are severely injured (Erikson, 1976). Yet, in healthcare settings, it *should* be possible to avoid adding trauma to that already wrought by the wrath of illness or disease. Carol Ann spoke of "treatment by gang warfare" (a telling phrase for its insinuation of nearby urbanicity rather than distant, more global conflict) as if healthcare occurred in an armed and hostile environment. The phrase signals a subjugation of healthcare *and caring* to technocratic medical treatment. The knowledge and the power to change direction and be ambiguous obfuscate the loss in a manner reminiscent of childhood tales. Carol Ann's "What do I do? What do I do?"

and driving herself to the hospital was like stepping through Alice's looking glass; "Wonderland" has strange ways of making the familiar strange and the strange familiar (Sacks, 1985).

Aloneness is particularly fearful amidst a hubbub of activity, for it then whispers alienation on top of being vulnerable to a risk that cannot be pinned down but must be dealt with by oneself. Care behavior asserting detachment, impatience, and disinterest generates feelings of shame, anger, and fear (Drew, 1986), but the gluttonous "indulgence of technology" leaves professional integrity perpetually at risk for moral defection. Along with depersonalized care, rates of iatrogenic injury, liability, and stress catapult with increased complexity of and dependence on technology, as well as with endless cycles of new personnel (Sinclair, 1988). Patients become things, patients' problems are things; patients with wounds are things with things (Gadow, 1989). And wounds that convey the imagination to the internal body are particularly destabilizing, doing violence to symbols and meanings of bodies as integral and self-contained, knowable and predictable parts of the self (Haraway, 1992; Lupton, 1994).

Who's Who and Other Mysteries

The moral flaw in women's healthcare, according to many gender and justice scholars, is unequal access to services. The primary ethical issue may indeed be access, but not necessarily access to healthcare. An issue of equal importance is women's access to their experience, access to meanings that establish the woman at the center of her own health. (Gadow, 1994, p. 295)

Care relationships are far more perplexing than meet the eye, while each identified episode and category of need tends to be treated separately with no one in charge (Caines, 1997), save perhaps fiscal management. A deeply imbedded history of images and practices of professional autonomy and individualistic division of labor perpetuates asymmetrical and solo performances, as well as individuated responsibility, in spite of the standardized procedures and passive acceptance by practitioners of relationships and interactions with clients that echo the market economy (Kleinman, 1995). Given the composition of disengaged modern selfhood (Richardson, Rogers, & McCarroll, 1998), it may all be more daunting than acknowledged.

Carol Ann often experienced the trickle-down effect of clinicians who were unclear how best to do a nearly impossible job. The very shape of healthcare is changing as formal hierarchy is replaced, unevenly in spurts and lulls, by less centralized self-help, participatory democracy, and convoluted, ever-changing coalitions. Nurses, as the most persistently present members of the team, are expected to be vocal in their advocacy of patients (Zalumas, 1995), but real circumstances often preclude their readiness and opportunity to advocate. While relational narratives are constructed to make sense of ambiguous stories (Gadow, 1994), nursing practice frequently suffers in the hands of leadership focused on more concrete outcome-measuring tasks, such as laboratory or other medical results. With no real care relationship relating to ethical responsibilities beyond the immediate task, it is hardly surprising that collaboration between in-patient and out-patient care becomes even more nebulous.

In critical care settings, already withering communication is further submitted to transformation into talk *about* rather than *to* or *with* patients (Halm & Alpen, 1993). While patients were traditionally moralistically classified as "good" or "bad," often by the strength of their affirmation of the "good doctor" or "good nurse" image, the situation today is further confounded by various contending models within and between biomedical specialty world-views (Stein, 1990). "Good" patients, in addition to not being responsible for their disease conditions and their control, respond readily to treatment and are compliant "winners" in battles against disease (Lupton, 1994; Stein, 1990). And it is the biological pathology of disease that biomedicine teaches as authentic, not the "untrustworthy story of illness as experience" (Kleinman, 1995, p. 32).

Symbolic struggles for voice take cultural casualties. On hospital teams, the orchestration of collective performance emphasizes coalition formation over its conduct and outcomes. In attempts to predict and control outcomes, combinations of people collaborating in a healthcare setting are constantly changing, with "teams"—regardless of what takes place on paper—appearing, disappearing, and being co-configured in serial new forms, in response to complex and changing needs and often without a constant core (Engeström, Engeström, & Kärkkäinen, 1995). Control, responsibility, and trust are reconceptualized and redistributed, essentially being rechoreographed in endless improvisation in response to changes in sociohistorical conditions and always with spatial, temporal, and ethical implications.

Cries from patients imploring to be listened to are hardly new (e.g.,

"Foreigner," 1912; Hanson, 1916; Haybach, 1993). But nursing care in a capitalistic system is compromised by sanction of an ethic dictating that caring is an option that comes last, as if it were something superfluous. Despite the complexity of patient status, it was Carol Ann's experience that someone who is both a patient and a health professional was treated differently from others who are not both. Collegiality remained confusing and uncomfortably stratified. Presence and connecting were fogged, and responsibility likewise blurred, in ways reminiscent of claims that institutional policy is designed to prevent closeness with patients (Cohen et al., 1994). But to Carol Ann, given her conviction that "they" control, losing her connection with "them" meant to her that she was losing control.

Carol Ann feared that her professional credentials negatively influenced her treatment and care. Perhaps that response is a consequence of the argument that Carol Ann sought something, a skill of involvement (Benner, Stannard, & Hooper, 1996) that only expert professional carers typically give. Carol Ann had impressive credentials, but nurses and nursing supplemental personnel changed work locations so often that few knew much about Carol Ann's background. At various times during her hospitalization, I talked with former students when I encountered them assigned to Carol Ann on the transplant unit. Unfortunately, none of them regularly worked that unit. Carol Ann got to know some regular staff and some even depended on her to help them solve problems with other patients' challenges. Most knew her as a hard taskmaster; Carol Ann's history with diabetes, and her knowledge of the fragility of her immune system and healing resources, led her to be a critical and defensive consumer. On the other hand, credentials seemed not so much to intimidate care providers as tempt them to slack off with care because someone like Carol Ann could tell them when something was truly needed. Her credentialing did not make Carol Ann a less-cared-about patient, although perhaps at times she may have been less cared for. Technicians knew they could depend on her to do some of the assessments and work they usually did and often to do it better. However, physicians less often recognized the value of either her learned or experiential knowledge or utilized it. Such a lack of acknowledgment is always painful, and it was to Carol Ann. As painful as being invalidated is to start with, the dynamic takes on new wounding power when the expertise might affect needed treatment and is trivialized by the socially recognized experts.

From Carol Ann's perspective, there was an assumption of collusion in relating to her "differently than they would if she were not a health professional." Yet there was also a difference in the relationship. Carol Ann: "You ask about '*they.*' Am I who I thought I was? One of them? They control; when the only other option is doing nothing, they surely have the control." This control affronted someone who felt vulnerable yet had seasoned knowledge about what is supposed to be a healing place. Carol Ann became preoccupied with such a need for vigilance on her own behalf that it haunted her every patient-care interaction and plagued her rest with dis-ease. The lay literature imparts numerous cautionary tales asserting every need for vigilance (for example, Boodman, 1996). Popular tips for prospective patients on choosing a hospital and checking out one's surgeon; knowing one's rights; trusting one's instinct; and checking and rechecking every drug, label, name, and test that comes along have extended beyond the purview of professional healthcare education and advanced practice experience. How is it, then, that an experienced consumer who lived intimately with and in the professional healthcare system for nearly all of her memorable life feared that "only 'nice neat patient patients' are cared about as well as cared for," and that the others are likely to be labeled "noncompliant" and "difficult," and to be punished for the audacity of self-assertion?

That disconcerting denying of who Carol Ann was, a painful claiming that she was someone she did not see herself to be, was part of the discourse on otherness (Harrison 1995; Kavanagh, 1988, 1991). Since only empathic engagement with others can result in moral sharing or even the understanding of others' suffering (Charmaz, 1999; Lévinas, 1988; Peperzak, Critchley, & Bernasconi, 1996), selective disinterest and recognition of who the other is alleviates whole areas of responsibility. But Carol Ann's concern did not stop there and was transposed with leaden gravity to everyday practice: If who and what she was could be so nonchalantly misread, "what of doctors' orders?" Carol Ann's personal identity was integrally one of an expert and experienced critical care nurse. Even as that identity was eroded and painfully relinquished in her posttransplant years, Carol Ann wanted to be proud of her profession. Not only did she not want to be that "oops" of failure, she wanted her high standards to be generalized enough to prevent other "oops" situations.

Nurses are caught in the tension of trying to care for people in a society that essentially refuses to value caring (Reverby, 1987a), for it is treating and curing that *matter* in a science-dazzled culture. While patient-centered bioethics are not invisible in biomedicine, the orientation is not a highly valued one (Kleinman, 1995). Care relationships, to say nothing of *caring* relationships, are costly luxuries. Care providing and care receiving, like critical pathways, are solutions to particular sets of historical problems internal to specific institutions. The problem is the contradiction created between normative and linear sequences of procedures and superseding ever more encompassing configurations of needs.

Another thing that *mattered* to Carol Ann was who she is, her cultural orientation to being American *and* African American (West, 1993). The consequences of healthcare providers' slipshod inattentiveness to how patients and families perceive and use their own personal and cultural orientations, as well as to how clinicians use the patient's culture, are well documented (Capers, 1985; Jezewski, 1993; Kavanagh, 1988, 1991; Kavanagh & Kennedy, 1992; Kleinman, 1988b; Leininger, 1991; Lipson & Steiger, 1996; Milio, 1970; Ory, Simons, Verhulst, Leenders, & Wolters, 1991; Pedersen, 1985; Pinderhughes, 1982; Stein, 1985). Carol Ann's realization that her chart for months contained a mistaken assumption of her identity as a "41 year old white woman" was, to her, akin to "treating the wrong patient" (Devereux, 1956). Such distressing communicative rupture is symptomatic of failure to take into account the real and local worlds in which people live and its links with suffering and disruption of personal identity, including race and ethnicity.

It is difficult to hear views and to understand ways that differ from those of one's own orientation, but the portentous alternatives are stereotyping and mislabeling. Race in the U.S.A. must be understood as a nexus of social relationships that perpetuate oppressive power relations between populations presumed to be essentially different (Harrison, 1995; Spelman, 1997). Practices need not be intentional to be construed as racist. When one's life is lived in a society in which race continues to be significant on many levels, there is a contradictory reality in not having one, of being neither black nor white (or both) in a social

organization normally beset with ruthlessly clear-cut bureaucratic classi-
fying and categorizing. In Carol Ann's case, race and ethnicity also spoke
to choice, commitment, and sense of self. She was proud of her ethnic
and racial heritage and focused a studious and attentive eye on family
stories and the rich genealogical details of her ancestry. Multicultural-
ism was not to her something anti-American or given to politically safe
"superchunking" into culture-minimizing larger groups (Rush, 1996),
but a promise of exploring and sharing meaningful commonalties and
differences. No matter how threatened her body may have been, the
struggle for self included, for Carol Ann, the cultural self (Rumann,
1998). In addition to the medical situation she faced and, with it, the
sense of loss of professional identity and community, for Carol Ann another level of trauma was inflicted by what she saw as racial and ethnic
mislabeling. While some may not have considered that especially significant, to Carol Ann it mattered *deeply*.

One might ask what difference more caring might have made to
Carol Ann, or even whether one can ever have enough of it. Many patients do not have the caring expressed to them from family and friends
that Carol Ann had; she was blessed, and she said so often. She also
worked hard at relationships to make and keep them caring. But even
with all of that caring, Carol Ann longed for something more. She
wanted someone(s) who knew well her medical situation, someone(s)
*with the status and authority of the healthcare professions and from
inside the organization* to know and alleviate her desperate need for
vigilance, her sense of powerlessness and vulnerability, her pain, and her
aloneness with her myriad life-threatening events and her catastrophic
illness. Although most health professionals have not personally experienced the problems their clients experience, they can and often do have
an intimacy with those experiences that goes beyond the empathy, sympathy, and compassion of the most sensitive friend or family member.

Carol Ann wanted to experience people "being there" in that sense
and in that role, and she wanted that experience to extend to all aspects
of her needs and care. She experienced a need to trust them to be there,
not as empathic and compassionate friends such as myself who may
have knowledge that was relevant but, no matter how committed, had
no obligation beyond personal relationship. Nor did it matter to her
whether or not they had experiences similar to hers, although, ideally,
she wanted to know that they were *sharing* her difficulties and fears as

if they had a relationship with the problem just as extensive and vital as her own. The crucial constituent, however, was her wanting and needing to know that they were there as dependable resources whose design and purpose it was to care for her when she needed them. There were two facets of this: Carol Ann, who prided herself on being an independent woman, could not justify making demands on anyone outside such a status, role, and function and resented having to do so from time to time in desperation; and she firmly believed that the failure of an organization to provide the caring she associated with such a resource (as well as the failure to even *hear* and acknowledge her repeated requests for same) represented a deficit in clinical reasoning, ethical comportment, and caring practice that she could neither forget nor forgive. In terms of outcomes, more caring (as recognized and experienced by Carol Ann) might not have prolonged her life a moment, impeded her physical decline, or speeded healing in any way. But it might have made her journey easier, less lonely, less fearful. As her father told me after Carol Ann's death, "The bottom line is that it might have made her situation more bearable for her." Sometimes that's all we can do, but it is no small thing, making sense of *the other's* suffering and pain.

It is a part of humanness to wonder about and try to make sense of our existence (Heidegger, 1962). Suffering is a moral experience (Charmaz, 1999; Kleinman, 1995) that is framed culturally as, paradoxically, something both to be avoided and essential to human growth (Rawlinson, 1986; Saunders, 1996). We hear often, "No pain, no gain." At the same time, suffering is profoundly social, helping as it does in constituting the social world (Kleinman, Das, & Lock, 1997). Essentially an individual's experience of threat to the self (Kahn & Steeves, 1986), suffering, as the experience of pain, involves the perceptions of wholeness, personhood, and self-identity (Cassell, 1991).

The meaning of suffering varies greatly (Kleinman et al., 1997; Steeves & Kahn, 1987) and can be manipulated (Steeves, 1992), masked, delayed, or rechanneled (Frank, 1992). Finding meaning in a situation can affect suffering (Frankl, 1972), yet there are aspects of pain and suffering for which there is no justification. Society grapples with the failure to bring together the mechanistic views of science, ideas of "life force and therapeutic powers within patients" (Kleinman, 1995, p. 36), more holistic convictions, and economical concerns (Boschma, 1994; Capra, 1982; Davis-Floyd & St. John, 1998; Lyng, 1990). Hahn (1995) pointed out that physicians do not generally bridge the gap between themselves and patients until commonalties occur that bring the physician into patienthood to recognize his or her own suffering, fear, and needs, and the need for experiences to be lived rather than managed (Frank, 1991; Gadamer 1996). But given the complex interrelationships among grief, suffering, compassion, trivialization, sympathy, and care (Spelman, 1997), it is not surprising that pleading for empathy from healthcare providers is not a new phenomenon (English, 1983).

While biomedicine obscures suffering by constructing medical realities and entifying them as diseases (Kleinman, 1995), physical pain is held by some to be the human experience both "most private" and "least communicable" (Arendt, 1959, p. 46). Humans both hope to be spared suffering (B. J. Good, 1994) and tend to be ambivalent about it. A lack of voice nearly always characterizes the interpersonal and cultural context within which suffering occurs (Morris, 1997), which has prompted the recommending of storytelling for exploring ideas around ethical concerns (Benner, 1991). In terms of understanding and acknowledging suffering, one wonders what might happen if bioethics paid serious attention to patients' stories (Morris, 1998).

Diabetics, unlike most healthcare professionals, learn from experience to trust their understandings of how their bodies work. Although it has been said that "[o]ne may metaphorically substitute the narrative for the body of the patient as the object of clinical scrutiny" (P. Atkinson, 1995, p. 149), Carol Ann felt her story was unheard, just as her knowledge about her body was ignored, until she put her resistance, designed to promote time and safety to heal, in *financial terms*. The political economy of late 20th-century healthcare bought her time through reprieves from medical attention that allowed her suffering to lessen.

Multiple versions of understanding tend to be viewed by biomedicine as more perplexing than enriching. In everyday life, health providers protect themselves against subjective experiences of body and spirit by learning early to objectify those patients' bodies. Collective objectification in a shared version of what is going on buffers pain inflicted in providing care or treatment that requires dissociating from one's own body to avoid suffering the other's pain (Gadow, 1989; Tisdale, 1986). The sufferer may be alienated (Younger, 1995), but pain is held at bay by carers. When distancing becomes a coping strategy, responsibility is shifted but not necessarily to other care takers as much as back to private ownership of the "problem" by the patient. There is solace in learning through professional socialization ("technocratic initiation" [Davis-Floyd & St. John, 1998]) that patients and their needs should not be coddled and patronized. There are few alternatives that are not overwhelming. Too much caring has been compared with opening the heart (Campo, 1996).

While carers as patients are said to experience analogous situations (Hahn, 1985), assigning Carol Ann a clear patient role required a wider gap than she felt needed to be. She was left struggling with only a defensive use of her knowledge and wondering how she could be and act as one of *them* and not so much as the patient, that different *other*. What is being a patient if not being *different* and *other*? Whether objectively flawed or empathically understood, patient-*is*-different. Although historical and contemporary caretaking often assumes and involves active roles on the parts of care recipients (Russell et al., 1997), it is usually clear who is providing care and who is *receiving* care (Griffin, 1983). Take, for instance, the pithy description by an anonymous nurse of her experience as a maternity patient that begins, " 'There is one thing you must remember,' the doctor told me, 'you are no longer a nurse. From now on you are a patient.' " ("A nurse goes . . . ," 1933, p. 845). But where is caring in this hierarchical role distinction that sacrifices possibilities for connecting, in minimizing risk of pain? Superficial friendliness mollifies powerful distancing in providing care. There is an insinuated gifting in the care and a stating that duty has been done. It is as if the ethics require one to ask: Is this enough to be fair and respectful? If the answer is yes, or if one is too busy or too tired to ask the question, any attempt may be "enough."

The body is said to "remember its pain, and 'fear' [is] the name given to this memory" (Young, 1997, p. 258). Although preliminary research indicates that the amount of stress experienced during the renal transplant process and its sequelae is directly correlated with patient outcome, quality of life is generally expected to improve after transplantation (Fallon et al., 1997). However, Carol Ann's experience was, to her, an anomaly of prolonged doubt, suffering, and unmet need. Although it is characteristic of biomedicine to construct "the object of therapeutic work without legitimating suffering" (Kleinman, 1995, p. 32), it is also quick to medicalize psychophysiological effects of suffering associated with trauma and extreme conditions with labeling such as Post-

Traumatic Stress Syndrome (PTSD) (Kleinman, 1995). It has long been known that the longer a traumatic situation is sustained, the more likely suffering is to be experienced with those events (Stouffer, 1949). Carol Ann communicated (sometimes even using associated terms such as "fighting," "doing battle," and "warfare") experiencing something like battle fatigue. She spoke often of suffering, which she variously described as psychological, existential, or spiritual, as well as physical.

Despite her experiencing and expressing the intense fear, helplessness, and recurrent dreams characteristic of PTSD, Carol Ann's providers' medicocentrism precluded recognition of her emotional and spiritual needs as significant. Despite six major surgeries and 8 months on the acute side of the transplant unit, potential support was preempted with offhand advice that she should let out a single scream and all would be well. Kleinman, a physician, points out that physicians are no more educated to face suffering that cannot be reversed than they are to limit the use of powerful technology. "Indeed suffering is converted into technical problems that transmogrify its existential roots" (Kleinman, 1995, p. 34). Since, in cultures of fear, repression systematically silences people through suffering (Kleinman, 1995), biomedicine's potential for sustaining such cultural traits is in itself unsettling and contradictory.

Embodiment: More Than a Patient's Casing

"Our bodies are the homes in which we live and provide us access to the world" (Saunders, 1996, p. 101). With transplantation, Carol Ann's body's workings become less coordinated, more fragmented, and more self-conscious. There are moral and emotional responses to such upheaval. Being human assumes that the body reflects, somehow, the state of the soul (White, 1991). When breakdown occurs in the skilled know-how of familiar, everyday living (Heidegger, 1962), practices and activities show up differently (Steeves & Kahn, 1995). The body remains omnipresent, albeit altered, demanding to be reckoned with as part of who and what we are. A lack of simple consideration and respect in healthcare interaction takes on powerful, potentially painful dimensions.

Cultural changes conspire against adequate recognition of the meaning of embodiment in practice. In the contemporary orientation toward wellness (Stein, 1990; Wolszon, 1998; Woods et al., 1988), any serious illness poses questions about the deepest sense of self in relation to embodied existence. Gone are the days when physiological anomalies more likely elicited scorn or sympathy than intervention strategies. New or changing health problems and their chronicity compound the situation with a sense of responsibility for being healthy.

In contrast to understandings rooted in science, embodiment is a lived experience by which Carol Ann had, over her years of socialized living, assigned characteristics to her body that changed as the situation did (Dreyfus, 1987; Merleau-Ponty, 1962). Her body, then, was not a foundation for concrete reality but a combining of "discursive processes, practices and physical matter" (Lupton, 1994, p. 49) that related symbiotically and symbolically with society. In other words, her existence being embodied (Gadow, 1994), Carol Ann's body was her vehicle for expressing her specific social reality (Price, 1993; Steeves & Kahn, 1995). Due to her parents' patient normalizing, that reality included a relationship with her diabetic body as her normal-for-her body (McWilliam, Stewart, Brown, Desai, & Coderre, 1996). After transplantation, however, that orientation no longer adequately fit the situation. The body that could be overlooked when it functioned normally, which for Carol Ann meant "normally diabetically," needed to be openly addressed in the changed situation involving end stage renal disease and transplantation. But, for Carol Ann, among those who provided her healthcare and who were most physically and intimately involved with her body, there was no one who addressed the colossal challenge she faced when the nature of her body changed and her sense of normative bodily wholeness was lost.

Carol Ann gained a functioning kidney but found she had, overall, been neither fine-tuned nor overhauled for the idealized, better-working physical self. Instead, she faced serial problems without apparent end. No longer a woman whose body happened to be diabetic and to have lapsed into renal failure, she realized that for the rest of her life she would be a "transplant patient." To Carol Ann, the "peculiar" meaning and cultural relevancy of the label implied a new and chronic role as a container for the new-to-her, successfully functioning kidney.

Carol Ann, musing one rainy day more than a year posttransplant:

My transplanted being has been so altered from my "original" diabetic body that what it means to *be* in relation to others in my social and cultural groups is different as well. Others see me as a courageous but chronically ill woman with an uncertain future and physical limitations. I don't necessarily see myself in those terms, but maybe here is where my hopes and expectations about who I am *now* (in contrast to prior to the transplant) merge. Am I fundamentally different due to the care experience I had or did not have? Although I perceive myself as a different being, I'm not sure I can describe what makes the transplanted being different from the diabetic being, except through the level and intensity of care required for the transplanted being and the realization that one can *never go back* to "simply" being diabetic. The kidney portion is finished, yet it's always in my mind as I work toward a situation more like my presurgical status.

Carol Ann's embodied practical knowledge, providing a sense of salience with skilled embodied know-how and practical reasoning in everyday, taken-for-granted living in and understandings of the world (Steeves & Kahn, 1995), retreated in desperation to hyper-vigilance. Under siege by time-pressured, compromised care and even carelessness, her watchful wariness defended against invasions of bodily boundaries, a diminishing sense of self, and a threatened withholding of part of her reality. She was convinced that she was perceived not as an embodied human being but as a patient whose body functioned as a casing for a kidney.

One wonders why it was so difficult for her carers to see or acknowledge her distress, for what happened to Carol Ann was neither unknown nor unique. In post-renal transplant patients, significantly altered physical self and body images have been documented as typical products of immunosuppressive therapy and as producing in patients stress and anxiety nearly as pressing as the fear of organ rejection (Fallon et al., 1997). It has been said that our embodiment is so necessary a requirement of our social identification that it would be ludicrous to say "I have arrived and I have brought my body with me" (Turner, 1984, p. 8). But Carol Ann felt she was not acknowledged as a whole and embodied person but as if only her body had arrived. And, to Carol Ann, the experience of embodiment, the subjective experience of having a body, *mattered*.

Needing Caring, but Living With Being "The Other"

Compassion has been exiled in the west. Part of the flight from compassion has been an ignorance of it that at times borders on forgetfulness, at times on repression, and at times on a conscious effort to distort it, control it and keep it down. This exile of compassion leads to the poison and pain that become incarnated whenever people are treated unfairly. Who can number the victims, living and dead, of the exile of compassion, sacrifices of human flesh to all the gods that humanity worships ahead of compassion? (M. Fox, 1990, pp. 1–2)

Until the end of her days, after her prolonged transplantation hospitalization, Carol Ann endured odious dreams of being rehospitalized. Experiencing dreams differs from lived and imagined experience, yet dreams reconstruct real-life experience and re-story its meanings (Mullen, 1994). The stories we cannot forget reflect their importance in our lives. What little research that has been done with post-renal transplant patients indicates that organ rejection is the primary fear of patients (Fallon et al., 1997). Yet, in the hospital, Carol-Ann-as-patient feared organ rejection less than she feared that no one would come when she needed help. Carol-Ann-as-professional, meanwhile, lamented that the illusory nature of caring seemed to be acceptable and expectable there.

While care is not something specific to nursing or medicine (Jecker & Self, 1991), Carol Ann had quickly learned to discriminate between care, which is formally and mechanically provided, and caring, which is more elusive and cannot be routinized. In addition to clinicians bringing more biological disease models than understandings of illness experiences with them to the clinical encounter, there is the issue of real versus ideal medical practice (Davis-Floyd & St. John, 1998; Stein, 1990).

The need for compassion and caring in modern care settings has not gone unnoticed by nursing leadership. Gradually, more attention has been given to caring and healing (for example, Gaut & Boykin, 1994). One effort to establish alternatives to contested paths and behavior-based realities, and to encourage understanding and caring, has been the use of storytelling as a pathway similar to other clinical pathways and group storytelling as a mechanism for communication sharing during the traditional rounds (Sarosi & O'Connor, 1993). Most research, however, continues to emphasize either mechanical and procedural practices or theoretical and philosophical discussion (Daniel, 1998; Griffin, 1983), which, although helpful for identifying needs, often leave strategies for implementable *caring practices* implicit and elusive. Without recognizing actual Concernful Practices, *caring* remains the too rare largess of those carers who are empathic, creative, and not harried beyond the point of being able to be caring, as well as able to provide care (Diekelmann, 1994–1999, 2001; Kavanagh, Absalom, Beil, & Schliessmann, 1999; Levine, 1973/1997).

For decades, Carol Ann's lifestory was one of controlling the self so that disease merely shaped but did not determine the paths of making choices and defining herself. Later she struggled to find health beyond the emotional, physical, and moral burdens of experiencing symptoms. There was a hidden cultural dialogue about self-reliance, dependency, self-respect, and being ill and wondering what was happening (Frank, 1991). Carol Ann asked more than once, "*How sick am I?* I wonder how sick I really am now that everything is so different and I can't tell. It's really hard to know myself anymore."

For Carol Ann, frustration and suffering were heightened by expectations for control when the body performed as a dense *other,* rather than as the familiar, readable, embodied knower and teller. Then there was contending with the false systems of public and private shame and blame, the sense of moral responsibility that modern Western cultures link to staying well and being self-reliant (Rawlinson, 1986). Tussling with basic issues that must be faced in every daily mass of medications and clinic appointments allowed putting off broader points of ethics and rights and justice.

Carol Ann's transition was painful. She resisted marks of disability: the wheelchair shopping cart, the handicapped sticker for parking, a cane. She trusted herself less as a driver. There was an insidious awareness of the chronicity of her new health status that germinated and grew unbidden. Like a powerful weed in the garden, or a strong but toneless voice in the choir, it could not be overlooked or put aside. Carol Ann's life continued to be shaped by the transplant experience. Transplantation and diabetic sequelae merged and seemed to mass collective strength. She resented medical intervention, the meaning of which she could no longer relate to her familiar diabetic self, that seemed to contribute more to her suffering than its alleviation. So much was out of control that nearly any predictability became something to hang on to and to preserve. The reality of limited capacity to know, predict, and control life events and problems, even those as profound as suffering and dying, are always part of, never apart from everyday living. It seemed superficial to recount the loss of function that led to reconsideration of life meanings and social status (Katz & Florian, 1986–87), for Carol Ann believed that, in real life, it was picking up and moving on that required her energies. Meanwhile, the insurance company pressed for decisions: "'You either return to work or you are permanently disabled.' I am permanently disabled. But I am not really sure I accept it, even though an official decision has been made."

Carol Ann tried writing in her journals, when she had the energy, to allay some of "the ghosts." Many things remained unresolved, but she found that reflecting on them "helps bring them to the surface and I can write about them." Carol Ann valued the opportunities she had for "making memories." She tried to maintain her church involvement but found herself unable to plan and live day by day, which was a frustrating situation for such an organized woman. She found herself paying more attention "to relationships, doing things with friends, having a relaxing home." She enjoyed making personalized greeting cards on her computer. But, at the same time, although she knew her participatory contributions to her church and a few other organizations, and her occasional professional ethical–legal consultation, were significant, she grieved their falling far short of the future she had envisioned. It was a future shortened in so many ways that she was "amazed that mornings come. You know, when you're circling the drain, you sort of feel like you have one foot in the grave and the other on a banana peel."

Carol Ann fought valiantly against being sick, protecting herself in every way she could, struggling to remain vigilant when the magnitude of both disease and treatment processes threatened defeat. She had the verve to do that. But part of suffering is feeling estranged, alienated, and alone—of not being known (Cassell, 1991) or not being part of the community one expects to be part of (Anderson, 1986; Seeman, 1983; Stokols, 1975). This can take on particularly ominous meaning for the chronically ill (Miller, 1985). For Carol Ann, the most acute alienation, the greatest sense of *otherness,* was from the healthcare community. Carol Ann experienced herself as an African American health professional, but it became a struggle to maintain that identity when she was so much a patient in the care of others and was viewed as such by those others, some of whom did not know her and did not try to know her deeply.

I don't fit the categories when the alumni group wants to know about current position and employer. I wonder if being a professional and feeling helpless make you especially powerless as a patient, particularly when being a patient is a full-time job.

Carol Ann became less future-oriented than she had been.

"I am not promised tomorrow" has new meaning for me. It is not the "what" that happens but the accumulation of many unpredictable "whats." I fear some-times that the bottle is filling up and an extra drop will make it spill over.

Time allowed some healing by distancing the trauma and "changing relationships with details so that the pain is altered, just as time has altered the pain I experienced in my youth when I used old insulin needles in a petite body." She valued the distancing of emotional pain she felt watching her parents "suffer my pain." But what she called a "cloud of temporariness" hung over everything, despite the pervading, parallel, and perhaps seemingly contradictory oppression of chronicity.

Carol Ann was told to expect her cadaver transplant to last 5 to 7 years, at best. Then the surgeon, behaving as if a subsequent transplant was assumed, said, "Next time I would like it to be living donor." Carol Ann wholeheartedly resented not being asked to give consent for specu-lating about "next time," that it was taken for granted. Ominously bur-dened by another new expectation, Carol Ann expressed her feelings to the physician. His response was, "There will be some way to get you to come around."

Could this be a final, "extra drop"? The insidious strain snowballed until she retreated into a conscious effort to limit her attention to the past and present. "I reflect on what *has* happened; it's better not to dwell on the future." Agreeing wholeheartedly that "a patient needs emotionally, morally, to be recognized for what he [*sic*] was and hopes to become again" (Griffin, 1983, p. 291), Carol Ann decided that she could no longer afford to look ahead.

I never doubted this transplant. I did not want to die. I do not want to die! But I don't know if I could say yes to another transplant after all this. I really don't think I could do that.

Her sense of dispiriting in-betweenness, of being neither here nor there, imposed a kind of invisibility on Carol Ann. Her sense of self-renewal was damaged, despite unflagging support from family and friends. She experienced her care as both conflicted, for its symbolizing of thwarted hopes, and distanced, in its wanting of personal caring and connecting (Chesla, 1994). No one set about to do these things that way; they merely did not set about caring in other ways. The care was simply not profound, present, connecting, compassionate (in the sense of "suffering with" [Lane, 1987]), and *caring* enough to nurture the possibilities (Hanneman, 1996).

We talked about healing coming from within but being facilitated from without. But Carol Ann insisted, "It can't be jump-started like a battery. It has to be tenderly nurtured." That's where the caring mattered to her. Caring could facilitate healing, but it could not make it happen. Feeling unconnected and being mislabeled, Carol Ann experienced a sense of removal from the caring humanness of community, of being neither completely patient nor fully health professional, of feeling dependent and yet threatened with abandonment, with each of those being as victimized and exploited as the other. She was tagged as "black" or "white" according to careless jottings. While struggling to live a life, she felt unrecognized for who she thought she was and treated as if *it did not matter.*

Carol Ann was so much a nurse that I teased her about it being part of her DNA. She found refuge as well as identity in her professional socialization, experience, and credentials, which made it excruciatingly difficult for her to give it up to being "disabled." For the first 2 years posttransplant, she said she was going to write a companion article to go with this chapter. It would be written specifically for nurses. But every time she started writing, it came out sounding like a medical report—lab results, technical terms—and Carol-Ann-the-person and -the-patient "went missing" from the experience that Carol-Ann-the-professional reported. As a critical care nurse, Carol Ann knew and thought a lot about disease. As a patient, the experiential became more prominent, but the disease and critical care processes were still very important to her. Carol Ann reframed the facts of her experience as medical reports and then would sorely miss the caring she wanted from others who shared her critical care orientation when the cold hard medical facts were painfully ruthless.

Only in engaging with their patients can nurses and other healthcare providers ease suffering (Morse, Bottorff, Anderson, O'Brien, & Solberg, 1992), for suffering must be known and recognized if it is to be effectively treated (Cassell, 1991). For

. . . nothing cures me of my needs, and I've
Among my bitter medicines no salve
To calm my troubled, trembling soul.
        (Campo, 1996, *The Doctor*, p. 94)

While Carol Ann also felt increasingly apart from healthy and functional adults, she especially grieved for the loss of collegial membership as a healthcare provider. There is an irony in nursing's long ago setting its sights on the construct of caring as its raison d'être when, as a profession, it still cannot satisfactorily define what that is. In recent years, studies of actual *care practices* have done much to elucidate care, but caring remains elusive. Yet there is "something out there" that we all need and long for and that we experience as caring—or as lack thereof. Some might call it love, but the confusion that term engenders is acceptable to neither the culture of the scientific community nor the discipline. Carol Ann knew nursing's continued grappling with some basic unknowns as she explored her own experience of not experiencing adequate caring and the need for recognizing that even the best textbook care cannot fill a patient's need for caring. She knew it involves, somehow, a connecting on a deeper level of humanity. And she held nursing more accountable than other healthcare disciplines for both caring and lack of caring. "*Nursing* roles are supposed to be *about* caring." It is not the same caring that a father shares, or a close friend, but it is something that (ideally) transcends the mechanical provision of basic care, even when delivered with a smile. Carol Ann believed that nurses should be able to share the patient's situation in ways that others (even those who care deeply about the ill individual) cannot. Caring nurses do not replace those others, but (again, ideally) they assist patients in negotiating illness (or other problems or experiences) in special ways. Caring is about both freedom and obligation (Sartre & Levy, 1996) that lead to humanness on personal and collective levels. But is it most immediately about connecting for restoring the worlds of care and compassion for those with pain, if *caring* is to be? "But the eyes are blind. One must look with the heart . . ." (Saint-Exupéry, 1943, p. 82).

What would Carol Ann want others to gain from her story? In the simplest terms, she longed for a narrowing of that gap between critical illness as it is understood by someone experiencing it and the meaning it holds for those who care for such patients. This symbolized, to Carol Ann, interrelationships between ethics and context for which she held all healthcare professionals responsible. But hers is, at least in part, a story of breakdown in ethical clinical reasoning (Benner et al., 1999) and that of dependence on procedurally guided conclusions that failed both to protect Carol Ann and to prevent further breakdown. The story does not end there, however. Although Carol Ann held the many physicians involved in her treatment accountable for hegemonic manipulations that stripped her of much of her identity, self-esteem, and, at times, basic human dignity, it is surely significant that there was so little evidence of nurses interceding on her behalf.

When she felt up to it, Carol Ann was not above "inquisitioning" nurses (and physicians when they would tolerate it) about their interpretations of their roles. She inevitably gloomily reported scant if any signs of relating to practice, either theoretical or applied, that extended beyond technical reasoning. Given Carol Ann's commitment to moral reasoning in clinical situations (a cross-cultural exploration of nurses, which was the focus of her dissertation), there is a special sadness in her own story in which physicians could not, would not, or otherwise did not hear her—and the nurses were not caring enough to glean this oft-stated need, which to Carol Ann loomed like a wound left unsutured, and the dynamics involved to insist that the gap be closed. Her journey would still have been arduous, but it might have been a little "more bearable." The actuality of that unhealed wound now unchangeable, Carol Ann would have liked her story to contribute to understanding and learning and for her message to be—finally—heard.

Epilogue

Like anxious parents, Carol Ann and I nurtured this chapter into something very close to its present shape over the 4 years after her transplant. During that time, her determination to regain her health "as a normal person with diabetes" was painfully replaced through a not fully successful struggle to recreate a positive identity as, first, a "transplant patient" and, then, a "transplant patient who is disabled." For Carol Ann, reframing her dreams about her role in nursing research and nursing education was an excruciating loss, and, with her diabetes increasingly unmanageable and unpredictable, eventually her father even had to lay it on the line about her no longer being able to drive.

She did not feel well during the holidays but was proud of meeting many of her commitments to her church, her friends, and her family. "This is all I can do. I have to get used to that. But I can do this." A few weeks later she discovered a sore on the bottom of one foot; she had not known it was there until she found "blood and gore all over the bottom of my sock" when she took it off one evening. The sore did not respond to medical intervention and, in February, 5 days after the sudden and unanticipated death of her mother, Carol Ann had a below-the-knee amputation. Several bouts of intensive care ensued and then what seemed to her a very long, depressing stint of recuperation in a nursing home. She could no longer negotiate the stairs to her apartment, so her father and some friends packed up her belongings and stored them for her in their basements and spare rooms. Finally, she moved into another apartment of her own in a sheltered living facility.

When I talked with her a few days after her move into her new home, Carol Ann was enthusiastic about walking with her prosthesis and spending less time in a wheelchair. She was still concerned about her father's having to deal with her mother's loss, and she was excited about the next day's trip with a small group to St. Michael's Island—"My first outing with the prosthesis! A trial run! Well, maybe not a run exactly, but no wheelchair!" I told her I was working on the chapter and that I was thrilled that she sounded so much better, "You know I can't publish this thing without you!" She laughed and said, "Oh, yes you can!" But she was eager to pursue the project, and we made plans for me to take her to several medical appointments during the following week. It had been some time since Carol Ann had the energy to read, critique, and add directly to the manuscript. We would use the time before and after the appointments to talk through changes so that we could most accurately reflect her experience. She wanted to be sure her stories from the amputation were included, in particular one about her horror of hearing nurses making comments such as "Her pressure's dropping! She's dying! She's dying!" She could plainly hear them and could in no way overtly respond. That was in February.

In June, Carol Ann went on her day trip to St. Michael's and had a great time. She got a little queasy on the way home and decided she had "overdone a little." The next day the visiting nurse found her still feeling ill and suggested a trip to the hospital. Tests were run and Carol Ann was admitted, with DNR orders. She died a few hours later, a brave and loving 45-year-old woman with, according to the physician, "the veins of an eighty year old." Her father, the Reverend Shelby Rooks, told me "It was time. I'm sure she knew that too. She has suffered terribly ever since the transplant and had diarrhea every single day—many times every single day—for these 4 years. How can anybody put up with that? Now she'll finally have some peace." He added later, "For Carol, dying was healing. Her body was disintegrating and needed to die in order that she be finally healed." We will never know the other stories that Carol Ann wanted to share, but we can bet they were about caring.

References

Aaronson, M. (1989, May/June). The case manager-home visitor. *Child Welfare, 68*, 339–346.

Adorno, T. W. (1973). *Negative dialectics* (E. B. Ashton, Trans.). New York: Continuum.

Allen, M. N., & L. Jensen. (1990). Hermeneutical inquiry—Meaning and scope. *Western Journal of Nursing Research, 12*, 241–253.

Anderson, L. (1986). A model of estrangement—Including a theoretical understanding of loneliness. *Psychological Reports, 58*, 683–695.

Arendt, H. (1959). *The human condition.* Garden City, NY: Doubleday-Anchor.

Ariès, P. (1981). *The hour of our death* (H. Weaver, Trans.). New York: Alfred A. Knopf. (Original work published 1977)

Asch, D. A., Shea, J. A., Jedrziewski, M. K., & Bosk, C. L. (1997). The limits of suffering: Critical care nurses' views of hospital care at the end of life. *Social Science and Medicine, 45*, 1661–1668.

Ashley, J. (1976). *Hospitals' paternalism and the roles of the nurse.* New York: Teacher's College Press.

Atkinson, P. (1995). *Medical talk and medical work: The liturgy of the clinic.* London: Sage.

Atkinson, R. (1995). *The gift of stories: Practical and spiritual applications of autobiography, life stories, and personal mythmaking.* Westport, CT: Bergin & Garvey.

Athay, S. (1993, December). Giving and getting. *American Demographics, 15*, 46–49.

Baer, H. A. (1987). *Encounters with biomedicine: Case studies in medical anthropology.* New York: Gordon & Breach Science.

Baillie, L. (1996). A phenomenological study of the nature of empathy. *Journal of Advanced Nursing, 24*, 1300–1308.

Barkauskas, V. H. (1983, May). Effectiveness of public health nurse home visits to primiparous mothers and their infants. *American Journal of Public Health, 73*, 573–580.

Barry, C. A., Britten, N., Barber, N., Bradley, C., & Stevenson, F. (1999). Using reflexivity to optimize teamwork in qualitative research. *Qualitative Health Research, 9*, 26–44.

Bartunek, J. M., & Louis, M. R. (1996). *Insider/outsider team research.* Thousand Oaks, CA: Sage.

Ben-Ari, A. T. (1995). It's the telling that makes the difference. In R. Josselson & A. Lieblich (Eds.), *Interpreting experience: The narrative study of lives* (pp. 153–172). Thousand Oaks, CA: Sage.

Benner, P. (1984). *From novice to expert: Excellence and power in clinical nursing.* Menlo Park, CA: Addison-Wesley.

Benner, P. (1991). The role of experience, narrative, and community in skilled ethical comportment. *Advances in Nursing Science, 14*, 1–21.

Benner, P., Hooper-Kyriakidis, P., & Stannard, D. (1999). *Clinical wisdom and interventions in critical care: A thinking-in-action approach.* Philadelphia: W. B. Saunders.

Benner, P., Stannard, D., & Hooper, P. L. (1996). A "thinking-in-action" approach to teaching clinical judgment: A classroom innovation for acute care advanced practice nurses. *Advanced Practice Nursing Quarterly, 1,* 70–77.

Benner, P., Tanner, C. A., & Chesla, C. A. (1996). *Expertise in nursing practice: Caring, clinical judgment, and ethics.* New York: Springer Publishing.

Benner, P., & Wrubel, J. (1989). *The primacy of caring: Stress and coping in health and illness.* Reading, MA: Addison-Wesley.

Beverley, J. (2000). Testimonio, subalternity, and narrative authority. In N. K. Denzin & Y. S. Lincoln (Eds.), *Handbook of qualitative research* (2nd ed., pp. 555–566). Thousand Oaks, CA: Sage.

Bloom, L. R. (1996). Stories of one's own: Nonunitary subjectivity in narrative representation. *Qualitative Inquiry, 2,* 176–197.

Boodman, S. G. (1996, March 26). Consumer Reports on Health: Surviving Your Hospital Stay: Tips on choosing a hospital and checking out your surgeon. *Washington Post* (Health Supplement)

Boschma, G. (1994). The meaning of holism in nursing: Historical shifts in holistic nursing ideas. *Public Health Nursing, 11,* 324–330.

Boykin, A., & Schoenhofer, S. O. (1991). Story as link between nursing practice, ontology, epistemology. *Image, 23,* 245–248.

Broom, D. H. (1991). *Damned if we do: Contradictions in women's healthcare.* North Sydney, New South Wales, Australia: Allen & Unwin.

Burgoon, J. K., Olney, C. A., & Coker, R. A. (1987, Fall). The effects of communicator characteristics on patterns of reciprocity and compensation. *Journal of Nonverbal Behavior, 11,* 46–165.

Caines, E. (1997, May 9). A health lesson I never wanted: Need for National Health Service reforms. *New Statesman, 16,* 24.

Campbell, J. C., & Bunting, S. (1991). Voices and paradigms: Perspectives on critical and feminist theory in nursing. *Advances in Nursing Science, 13,* 1–15.

Campo, R. (1996). *What the body told.* Durham, NC: Duke University Press.

Capers, C. F. (1985). Nursing and the Afro-American client. *Topics in Clinical Nursing, 7,* 11–17.

Capra, F. (1982). *The turning point: Science, society and the rising culture.* New York: Simon & Schuster.

Casey, E. (1991). *Spirit and soul: Essays in philosophical psychology.* Dallas, TX: Spring Publications.

Cassell, E. J. (1991, May/June). Recognizing suffering. *Hastings Center Report,* 24–31.

Charmaz, K. (1999). Stories of suffering: Subjective tales and research narratives. *Qualitative Health Research, 9,* 362–382.

Chesla, C. A. (1994). Parents' caring practices with schizophrenic offspring. In P. Benner (Ed.), *Interpretive phenomenology: Embodiment, caring, and ethics in health and illness* (pp. 167–184). Thousand Oaks, CA: Sage.

Church, O. M. (1987). Historiography in nursing research. *Western Journal of Nursing Research, 9,* 275–279.

Cohen, M. Z., Hausner, J., & Johnson, M. (1994). Knowledge and presence: Accountability as described by nurses and surgical patients. *Journal of Professional Nursing, 10,* 177–185.

Cooper, M. C. (1991). Principle-oriented ethics and ethic of care: A creative tension. *Advances in Nursing Science, 14,* 22–31.

Corea, G. (1985). *The hidden malpractice: How American medicine mistreats women.* New York: Harper & Row.

Daniel, L. E. (1998). Vulnerability as a key to authenticity. *Image, 30,* 191–91.

Davis, A. J. (1981). Compassion, suffering, morality: Ethical dilemmas in caring. *Nursing Law and Ethics, 2,* 1–2, 6, 8.

Davis, D. (1991). Rich cases: The ethics of thick description. *Hastings Center Report, 21,* 12–17.

Davis, K. (1993). Nice doctors and invisible patients: The problem of power in feminist common sense. In A. D. Todd & S. Fisher (Eds.), *The social organization of doctor-patient communication* (pp. 243–265). Norwood, NJ: Ablex.

Davis-Floyd, R., & St. John, G. (1998). *From doctor to healer: The transformative journey.* New Brunswick, NJ: Rutgers University Press.

Denzin, N. K. (1997). *Interpretive ethnography: Ethnographic practices for the 21st century.* Thousand Oaks, CA: Sage.

Denzin, N. K., & Lincoln, Y. S. (2000). Introduction: The discipline and practice of qualitative research. In N. K. Denzin & Y. S. Lincoln (Eds.), *Handbook of qualitative research* (2nd ed., pp. 1–28). Thousand Oaks, CA: Sage.

Derrida, J. (1981). *Positions.* Chicago: University of Chicago Press.

Devereux, G. (1956). The wrong patient. *Therapeutic education.* New York: Harper.

DeVisser, P. A. (1981). The effects of technology on critical care nursing practice. *Focus on Critical Care, 7,* 26–29.

Diekelmann, N. (1991). The emancipatory power of the narrative. In *Curriculum revolution: Community building and activism* (pp. 41–62). New York: National League for Nursing.

Diekelmann, N. (1994–1999). Nursing Institute for Heideggerian Hermeneutical Studies and Advanced Nursing Institute for Heideggerian Hermeneutical Studies, University of Wisconsin–Madison.

Diekelmann, N. (2001). Narrative pedagogy: Heideggerian hermeneutical analyses of the lived experiences of students, teachers and clinicians. *Advances in Nursing Science, 23*(3), 53–71.

Doolittle, N. D. (1994). A clinical ethnography of stroke recovery. In P. Benner (Ed.), *Interpretive phenomenology: Embodiment, caring, and ethics in health and illness* (pp. 211–254). Thousand Oaks, CA: Sage.

Drew, N. (1986). Exclusion and confirmation: A phenomenology of patients' experiences with caregivers. *Image, 18,* 39–43.

Dreyfus, H. (1987). Husserl, Heidegger and modern existentialism. In B. McGee (Ed.), *The great philosophers: An introduction to Western philosophy* (pp. 254–277). London: BBC Books.

Dreyfus, H. L., Dreyfus, S. E., & Athanasiou, T. (1986). *Mind over machine: The power of human intuition and expertise in the era of the computer.* New York: Free Press.

Ellis, C., & Bochner, A. P. (Eds.). (1996). *Composing ethnography: Alternative forms of qualitative writing.* Walnut Creek, CA: AltaMira Press.

Engeström, Y., Engeström, R., & Kärkkäinen, M. (1995). Polycontextuality and boundary crossing in expert cognition: Learning and problem solving in complex work activities. *Learning and Instruction, 5,* 319–336.

English, M. (1983). Ordeal: Remember me? I'm the patient—the reason why, why this hospital is here, why you're here. *Nursing, 83*(13), 35–43.

Epstein, J. (1995). *Altered conditions: Disease, medicine, and storytelling.* New York: Routledge.

Erikson, K. (1976). *Everything in its path.* New York: Simon and Schuster.

Fábrega, H., Jr. (1997). *Evolution of sickness and healing.* Berkeley: University of California Press.

Fagin, C. (1975). Nurses' rights. *American Journal of Nursing, 75,* 82.

Fallon, M., Gould, D., & Wainwright, S. P. (1997). Stress and quality of life in the renal transplant patient: A preliminary investigation. *Journal of Advanced Nursing, 25,* 562–570.

Feagin, J. R., Orum, A. M., & Sjoberg, G. (Eds.). (1991). *A case for the case study.* Chapel Hill: University of North Carolina Press.

Fisher, S. (1986). *In the patient's best interest: Women and the politics of medical decisions.* New Brunswick, NJ: Rutgers University Press.

Fisher, S. (1995). *Nursing wounds: Nurse practitioners, doctors, women patients and the negotiation of meaning.* New Brunswick, NJ: Rutgers University Press.

"Foreigner." (1912). Leaves from a patient's notebook. *American Journal of Nursing, 13,* 17–20.

Forrest, D. (1989). The experience of caring. *Journal of Advanced Nursing, 14,* 815–823.

Foucault, M. (1973). *The birth of the clinic.* New York: Pantheon.

Fox, M. (1990). *A spirituality named compassion and the healing of the global village, Humpty Dumpty and us.* San Francisco: HarperSan Francisco.

Fox, N. (1993). *Postmodernism, sociology and health.* New York: Open University Press.

Frank, A. W. (1991). *At the will of the body: Reflections on illness.* Boston: Houghton Mifflin.

Frank, A. W. (1992). The pedagogy of suffering: Moral dimensions of psychological theory and research with the ill. *Theory and Psychology, 4,* 467–485.

Frank, A. W. (1995). *The wounded storyteller: Body, illness, and ethics.* Chicago: University of Chicago Press.

Frankl, V. (1972). *Man's search for meaning.* New York: Pocket Books.

Fry, S. T. (1989). The role of caring in theory of nursing ethics. *Hypatia, 4,* 89–103.

Gadamer, H. G. (1996). *The enigma of health: The art of healing in a scientific age* (J. Gaiger & N. Walker, Trans.). Stanford, CA: Stanford University Press.

Gadow, S. (1988). Covenant without cure: Letting go and holding on in chronic illness. In J. Watson & M. Ray (Eds.), *The ethics of care and the ethics of cure: Synthesis in chronicity* (pp. 5–14). New York: National League for Nursing.

Gadow, S. (1989). Clinical subjectivity: Advocacy with silent patients. *Nursing Clinics of North America, 24,* 535–541.

Gadow, S. (1994). Whose body? Whose story? The question about narrative in women's healthcare. *Soundings, 77,* 295–307.

Gaut, D. A., & Boykin, A. (Eds.). (1994). *Caring as healing: Renewal through hope.* New York: National League for Nursing Press.

Gittelsohn, J., Shankar, A. V., West, K. P., Jr., Ram, R. M., & Gnywali, T. (1997, Summer). Estimating reactivity in direct observation studies of health behaviors. *Human Organization, 56,* 182–189.

Good, B. J. (1994). *Medicine, rationality, and experience.* Cambridge, England: Cambridge University Press.

Good, M.-J. D. (1998). *American medicine: The quest for competence.* Berkeley: University of California Press.

Griffin, A. P. (1983). A philosophical analysis of caring in nursing. *Journal of Advanced Nursing 8,* 289–295.

Groopman, J. (1997). *The measure of our days: New beginnings at life's end.* New York: Viking.

Gubrium, J. F., & Holstein, J. A. (2000). Analyzing interpretive practice. In N. K. Denzin & Y. S. Lincoln (Eds.), *Handbook of qualitative research* (2nd ed., pp. 487–508). Thousand Oaks, CA: Sage.

Gunby, S. S. (1996). The lived experience of nursing students in caring for suffering individuals. *Holistic Nursing Practice, 10,* 63–73.

Hahn, R. A. (1985). Between two worlds: Physicians as patients. *Medical Anthropology Quarterly, 16,* 87–98.

Hahn, R. A. (1995). *Sickness and healing: An anthropological perspective.* New Haven, CT: Yale University Press.

Hall, B. (1990). The struggle of the diagnosed terminally ill person to maintain hope. *Nursing Science Quarterly, 2,* 177–184.

Halm, M. A., & Alpen, M. A. (1993). The impact of technology on patients and families. *Nursing Clinics of North America, 28,* 443–457.

Halpern, R. (1984, January). Lack of effects for home-based early intervention? Some possible explanations. *American Journal of Orthopsychiatry, 54,* 33–42.

Halttunen, K., & Perry, L. (Eds.). (1999). *Moral problems in American life: New perspectives on cultural history.* Ithaca, NY: Cornell University Press.

Hancock, B. L., & Pelton, L. H. (1989, January). Home visits: History and functions. *Social Casework, 70,* 21–27.

Hanneman, S. K. (1996). Advancing nursing practice with a unit-based clinical expert. *Image, 28,* 331–337.

Hanson, E. (1916). The personal and impersonal nurse. *American Journal of Nursing, 16,* 404–408.

Haraway, D. (1992). The promises of monsters: A regenerative politics for inappropriate/d others. In L. Grossberg, C. Nelson, & P. Treichler (Eds.), *Cultural studies* (pp. 295–337). New York: Routledge.

Harris, A., Ryan, M. C., & Belmont, M. F. (1997). More than a friend: The special bond between nurses. *American Journal of Nursing, 97,* 37–39.

Harrison, F. V. (1995). The persistent power of "race" in the cultural and political economy of racism. *Annual Review of Anthropology, 24,* 47–74.

Hauerwas, S. (1979). Reflections on suffering, death and medicine. *Ethics in Science and Medicine, 6,* 229–237.

Haybach, P. J. (1993). Suddenly seeing me. *American Journal of Nursing, 93,* 96.

Heidegger, M. (1962). *Being and time.* New York: Harper and Row.

Hollway, W., & Jefferson, T. (1997). Eliciting narrative through the in-depth interview. *Qualitative Inquiry, 3,* 53–70.

Holmes, C. A., & Warelow, P. J. (1997). Culture, needs and nursing: A critical theory approach. *Journal of Advanced Nursing, 25,* 463–470.

Honderich, T. (Ed.). (1995). *The Oxford companion to philosophy.* Oxford, England: Oxford University Press.

Hultgren, F. H. (1994). Ways of responding to the call. In M. E. Lashley, M. T. Neal,

E. T. Slunt, L. M. Berman, & F. H. Hultgren (Eds.), *Being called to care* (pp. 17–36). Albany: State University of New York Press.

Husserl, E. (1970). *The idea of phenomenology.* Evanston, IL: Northwestern University Press.

Jackson, M. (Ed.). (1996). *Things as they are: New directions in phenomenological anthropology.* Bloomington: Indiana University Press.

Jackson, M. M., Rickman, L. S., & Pugliese, G. (1999). Pathogens, old and new: An update for cardiovascular nurses. *Journal of Cardiovascular Nursing, 13,* 1–22.

Jaffe, D. T. (1985). Self-renewal: Personal transformation following extreme trauma. *Journal of Humanistic Psychology, 25,* 99–124.

Jecker, N. S., & Self, D. J. (1991). Separating care and cure: An analysis of historical and contemporary images of nursing and medicine. *Journal of Medicine and Philosophy, 16,* 285–306.

Jezewski, M. A. (1993). Culture brokering as a model for advocacy. *Nursing and Healthcare, 14,* 78–85.

Joel, L. A. (1997). Nursing and the human condition. *American Journal of Nursing, 97*(5), 7.

Johnson, C. D., Wicks, M. N., Milstead, J., Hartwig, M., & Hathaway, D. K. (1998). Racial and gender differences in quality of life following kidney transplantation. *Image, 30,* 125–130.

Joralemon, D., & Fujinaga, K. M. (1996). Studying the quality of life after organ transplantation: Research problems and solutions. *Social Science and Medicine, 44,* 1259–1269.

Josselson, R., & Lieblich, A. (Eds.). (1995). *Interpreting experience: The narrative study of lives.* Thousand Oaks, CA: Sage.

Kahn, D. L., & Steeves, R. H. (1986). The experience of suffering: Conceptual clarification and theoretical definition. *Journal of Advanced Nursing, 11,* 623–631.

Katz, S., & Florian, V. (1986–87). A comprehensive theoretical model of psychosocial reaction to loss. *International Journal of Psychiatry in Medicine, 16,* 325–345.

Kavanagh, K. H. (1988). The cost of caring: Nursing on a psychiatric intensive care unit. *Human Organization, 47,* 242–251.

Kavanagh, K. H. (1991). Invisibility and selective avoidance: Gender and ethnicity in psychiatry and psychiatric nursing staff interaction. *Culture, Medicine and Psychiatry, 15,* 245–274.

Kavanagh, K. H., Absalom, K., Beil, W., & Schliessmann, L. (1999). Cultural competence and connecting in America: A Lakota example. *Advances in Nursing Science, 21,* 9–31.

Kavanagh, K. H., & Kennedy, P. H. (1992). *Promoting cultural diversity: Strategies for healthcare professionals.* Newbury Park, CA: Sage.

Keller, K. L., Flatten, E. K., & Wilhite, B. C. (1988, Winter). Friendly visiting as a means of informing homebound senior citizens of health-related community services. *Journal of Community Health, 13,* 231–240.

Kent, R. N., & Foster, S. L. (1977). Direct observation procedures: Methodological issues in naturalistic settings. In A. Ciminero, K. Calhoun, & H. E. Adams (Eds.), *Handbook of Behavioral Assessment.* New York: Wiley.

Kleinman, A. (1988a). *The illness narratives.* New York: Basic Books.

Kleinman, A. (1988b). *Rethinking psychiatry: From cultural category to personal experience.* New York: Free Press.

Kleinman, A. (1995). *Writing at the margin: Discourse between anthropology and medicine*. Berkeley: University of California Press.

Kleinman, A., Das, V., & Lock, M. (Eds.). (1997). *Social suffering*. Berkeley: University of California Press.

Knaack, P. (1984). Phenomenological research. *Western Journal of Nursing Research, 6*, 107–114.

Koch, T. (1995). Interpretive approaches in nursing research: The influence of Husserl and Heidegger. *Journal of Advanced Nursing, 21*, 827–836.

Kockelmans, J. J. (1975). Toward an interpretative or hermeneutic social science. *Graduate Faculty Philosophy Journal, 5*, 73–96.

Kohut, H. (1977). *The restoration of the self*. New York: International Universities Press.

Kvale, S. (1996). *InterViews: An introduction to qualitative research interviewing*. Thousand Oaks, CA: Sage.

Kvale, S. (1999). The psychoanalytic interview as qualitative research. *Qualitative Inquiry, 5*, 87–113.

Lane, J. A. (1987). The care of the human spirit. *Journal of Professional Nursing, 3*, 332–337.

Lapadat, J. C., & Lindsay, A. C. (1999). Transcription in research and practice: From standardization of technique to interpretive positionings. *Qualitative Inquiry, 5*, 64–86.

Lawler, J. (1993). *Behind the screens: Nursing, somology, and the problem of the body*. Redwood City, CA: Benjamin/Cummings Publishing.

Leininger, M. M. (Ed.). (1991). *Culture care diversity and universality: A theory of nursing*. New York: National League for Nursing Press. (Pub. No. 15–2402).

Leitko, T. A., & Peterson, S. A. (1982). Social Exchange in Research: Toward a "New Deal" (Participatory Research). *The Journal of Applied Behavioral Science, 18*, 447–462.

Leonard, V. W. (1989). A Heideggerian phenomenologic perspective on the concept of the person. *Advances in Nursing Science, 11*(4), 40–55.

Lévinas, E. (1988). Useless suffering. In R. Bernagconi & D. Wood (Eds.), *The provocation of Lévinas* (pp. 79–96). London: Routledge.

Levine, M. E. (1997). On creativity in nursing. *Image, 29*, 216–217. (Originally published 1973)

Linde, C. (1993). *Life stories: The creation of coherence*. New York: Oxford University Press.

Lipson, J. G., & Steiger, N. J. (1996). *Self-care nursing in a multicultural context*. Thousand Oaks, CA: Sage.

Lister, P. (1997). The art of nursing in a "postmodern" context. *Journal of Advanced Nursing, 25*, 38–44.

Lock, M. (1997). Displacing suffering: The reconstruction of death in North America and Japan. In A. Kleinman, V. Das, & M. Lock (Eds.), *Social suffering* (pp. 207–244). Berkeley: University of California Press.

Lomnitz, L. A. (1988). Informal exchange networks in formal systems: A theoretical model. *American Anthropologist, 90*, 42–55.

Lowenberg, J. S. (1992). *Caring and responsibility: The crossroads between holistic practice and traditional medicine*. Philadelphia: University of Pennsylvania Press.

Lupton, D. (1994). *Medicine as culture: Illness, disease and the body in Western society*. London: Sage.

Lyng, S. (1990). *Holistic health and biological medicine.* Albany: State University of New York Press.

Lynn, J., & Teno, J. M. (1993). After the patient self-determination act: The need for empirical research on formal advance directives. *Hastings Center Report, 23,* 20–24.

Marshall, P. A. (1992). Anthropology and bioethics. *Medical Anthropology Quarterly, 6,* 49–73.

Martin, E. (1987). *The woman in the body: A cultural analysis of reproduction.* Boston: Beacon.

Mattingly, C. (1994). The concept of therapeutic "emplotment." *Social Science and Medicine, 38,* 811–822.

McLaughlin, T. (1996). *Street smarts and critical theory: Listening to the vernacular.* Madison: University of Wisconsin Press.

McWilliam, C. L., Stewart, M., Brown, J. B., Desai, K., & Coderre, P. (1996). Creating health with chronic illness. *Advances in Nursing Science, 18,* 1–15.

Mead, M. (1956). Nursing—primitive and civilized. *American Journal of Nursing, 56,* 1001–1004.

Meeker, B. F. (1984). Cooperative orientation, trust and reciprocity. *Human Relations, 37,* 225–243.

Merleau-Ponty, M. (1962). *Phenomenology of perception* (C. Smith, Trans.). London: Routledge & Kegan Paul.

Messing, K. (1998). Hospital trash: Cleaners speak of their role in disease prevention. *Medical Anthropology Quarterly, 12,* 168–187.

Milio, N. (1970). *9226 Kercheval: The storefront that did not burn.* Ann Arbor: University of Michigan Press.

Miller, J. F. (1985). Assessment of loneliness and spiritual well-being in chronically ill and healthy adults. *Journal of Professional Nursing, 1,* 79–85.

Minick, P. (1995). The power of human caring: Early recognition of patient problems. *Scholarly Inquiry for Nursing Practice, 9,* 303–317.

Mishler, E. G. (1991). Once upon a time. . . . *Journal of Narrative and Life History, 1*(2&3), 101–108.

Moorhouse, M. F., Geissler, A. C., & Doenges, M. E. (1987). *Critical care plans: Guidelines for patient care.* Philadelphia: F. A. Davis.

Moos, R. H. (1984). *Coping with physical illness.* New York: Plenum Medical Book Company.

Morris, D. B. (1997). About suffering: Voice, genre, and moral community. In A. Kleinman, V. Das, & M. Lock (Eds.), *Social suffering* (pp. 25–45). Berkeley: University of California Press.

Morris, D. B. (1998). *Illness and culture in the Postmodern Age.* Berkeley: University of California Press.

Morse, J. M., Bottorff, J., Anderson, G., O'Brien, B., & Solberg, S. (1992). Beyond empathy: Expanding expressions of caring. *Journal of Advanced Nursing, 18,* 1354–1361.

Morse, J. M., Bottorff, J., Neander, W., & Solberg, S. (1991). Comparative analysis of conceptualizations and theories of caring. *Image, 23,* 119–126.

Morse, J. M., & Johnson, J. L. (1991). *The illness experience: Dimensions of suffering.* Newbury Park, CA: Sage.

Morse, J. M., Solberg, S. M., Neander, W. L., Bottorff, J. L., & Johnson, J. L. (1990). Concepts of caring and caring as a concept. *Advances in Nursing Science, 13,* 1–14.

Mullen, C. (1994). A narrative exploration of the self I dream. *Journal of Curriculum Studies, 26,* 253–263.

Noddings, N. (1991). Stories in dialogue: Caring and interpersonal reasoning. In C. Witherell & N. Noddings (Eds.), *Stories lives tell: Narrative and dialogue in education* (pp. 157–170). New York: Teachers College Press.

A nurse goes to the hospital. (1993) *American Journal of Nursing, 33,* 845–849.

Ohnuki-Tierney, E. (1994). Brain death and organ transplantation: Cultural bases of medical technology. *Cultural Anthropology, 35,* 233–242.

Olrik, A. (1992). *Principles for oral narrative research [Nogle Grundsæininger for Sagnforskning]* (K. Wolf & J. Jensen, Trans.). Bloomington: University of Indiana Press. (Original work published 1921)

Ory, F. G., Simons, M., Verhulst, F. C., Leenders, F. R. H., & Wolters, W. H. G. (1991). Children who cross cultures. *Social Science and Medicine, 32,* 29–34.

Palmer, R. E. (1969). *Hermeneutics: Interpretation theory in Schleiermacher, Dilthey, Heidegger, and Gadamer.* Evanston, IL: Schmidt.

Patton, M. Q. (1990). *Qualitative evaluation and research methods* (2nd ed.). Newbury Park, CA: Sage.

Pedersen, P. (Ed.). (1985). Handbook of cross-cultural counseling and therapy. Westport, CT: Greenwood Press.

Peperzak, A. T., Critchley, S., & Bernasconi, R. (Eds.). (1996). *Emmanuel Lévinas: Basic philosophical writings.* Bloomington: Indiana University Press.

Pinderhughes, E. (1982). Afro-American families and the victim system. In M. McGoldrick, J. K. Pearce, & J. Giordano (Eds.), *Ethnicity and family therapy* (pp. 108–122). New York: Guilford Press.

Price, M. J. (1993). Exploration of body listening: Health and physical self-awareness in chronic illness. *Advances in Nursing Science, 15,* 37–5.

Puka, B. (1990). The liberation of caring: A different voice for Gilligan's *Different Voice. Hypatia, 5,* 58–83.

Rafael, A. R. F. (1996). Power and caring: A dialectic in nursing. *Advances in Nursing Science, 19,* 3–17.

Rank, M. R., & LeCroy, C. W. (1983, July). Toward a multiple perspective in family theory and practice: The case of social exchange theory, symbolic interactionism, and conflict theory. *Family Relations, 32,* 441–448.

Rawlinson, M. C. (1986). The sense of suffering. *Journal of Medicine and Philosophy, 11,* 39–62.

Reed, P. G. (1991). Toward a nursing theory of self-transcendence: Deductive reformulation using development theories. *Advances in Nursing Science, 13,* 64–77.

Remen, R. N. (1996a, Spring). In the service of life. *Noetic Science Review,* 24–25.

Remen, R. N. (1996b). *Kitchen table wisdom.* New York: Putnam.

Reverby, S. (1987a). A caring dilemma: Womanhood and nursing in historical perspective. *Nursing Research, 36,* 5–11.

Reverby, S. M. (1987b). *Ordered to care: The dilemma of American nursing, 1850–1945.* Cambridge, England: Cambridge University Press.

Rew, L., Bechtal, D., & Sapp, A. (1993). Self-as-instrument in qualitative research. *Nursing Research, 42,* 300–301.

Richards, L. (1999). Qualitative teamwork: Making it work. *Qualitative Health Research, 9,* 7–10.

Richardson, F. C., & Fowers, B. J. (1998a). Social inquiry: A hermeneutic reconceptualization. *American Behavioral Scientist, 41,* 461–464.

Richardson, F. C., & Fowers, B. J. (1998b). Interpretive social science: An overview. *American Behavioral Scientist, 41,* 465–495.

Richardson, F. C., Rogers, A., & McCarroll, J. (1998). Toward a dialogical self. *American Behavioral Scientist, 41,* 496–515.

Riley, J. M., & Omery, A. (1996). The scholarship of a practice discipline. *Holistic Nursing Practice, 10,* 7–14.

Rubin, H. J., & Rubin, J. S. (1995). *Qualitative interviewing: The art of hearing data.* Thousand Oaks, CA: Sage.

Rumann, S. M. (1998). The struggle for cultural self: "From numb to dumb." In R. C. Chávez & J. O'Donnell (Eds.), *Speaking the unpleasant: The politics of (non) engagement in the multicultural education terrain* (pp. 186–196). Albany: State University of New York Press.

Running, A. (1994). Visit: A method of existential inquiry for the development of nursing knowledge. In P. L. Chinn (Ed.), *Advances in methods of inquiry for nursing* (pp. 134–146). Gaithersburg, MD: Aspen Publishers.

Running, A. F. (1996). "A measure of my days" critiqued by the oldest old. *Image, 28,* 71–74.

Rush, J. A. (1996). *Clinical anthropology: An application of anthropological concepts within clinical settings.* Westport, CT: Praeger.

Russell, C. K., Bunting, S. M., & Gregory, D. M. (1997). Protective care-receiving: The active role of care-recipients. *Journal of Advanced Nursing, 25,* 532–540.

Sacks, O. (1985). *The man who mistook his wife for a hatrack and other clinical tales.* New York: Simon and Schuster.

Sacks, O. (1995). *An anthropologist on Mars: Seven paradoxical tales.* New York: Vintage Books.

Saint-Exupéry, A. de. (1943). *The little prince.* San Diego: Harcourt Brace.

Sandelowski, M. (1997). Knowing and forgetting: The challenge of technology for a reflexive practice science of nursing. In S. E. Thorne & V. E. Hayes (Eds.), *Nursing praxis: Knowledge and action* (pp. 69–88). Thousand Oaks, CA: Sage.

Sarosi, G. M., & O'Connor, P. (1993). The microstory pathway of executive nursing rounds: Tales for living caring. *Nursing Administration Quarterly, 17,* 30–37.

Sartre, J-P., & Levy, B. (1996). *Hope now: The 1980 interviews.* Chicago: The University of Chicago Press.

Saunders, J. M. (1996). HIV/AIDS and suffering. In B. R. Ferrell (Ed.), *Suffering* (pp. 95–119). Sudbury, MA: Jones and Bartlett Publishers.

Schon, D. (1991). *Educating the reflective practitioner: Toward a new design for teaching and leaning in the professions.* San Francisco: Jossey-Bass.

Schutze, F. (1992). Pressure and guilt: The experience of a young German soldier in World War Two and its biographical implications. *International Sociology, 7,* 187–208, 347–367.

Schwartz, W. B. (1998). *Life without disease: The pursuit of medical utopia.* Berkeley: University of California Press.

Scott, D. (1992, July). Reaching vulnerable populations: A framework for primary service role expansion (Australia). *American Journal of Orthopsychiatry, 62,* 332–341.

Scott-Maxwell, F. (1968). *The measure of my days.* New York: Alfred A. Knopf.

Seeman, M. (1983). Alienation motifs in contemporary theorizing: The hidden continuity of the classic themes. *Social Psychology Quarterly, 46,* 171–184.

Siegler, M., & Osgood, H. (1973). The sick role revisited. *Hastings Center Studies, 1,* 41–58.

Silva, M. C., Sorrell, J. M., & Sorrell, C. D. (1995). From Carper's patterns of knowing to ways of being: An ontological philosophical shift in nursing. *Advanced Nursing Science, 18,* 1–13.

Sinclair, V. (1988). High technology in critical care. *Focus on Critical Care, 15,* 36–41.

Sontag, S. (1978). *Illness as metaphor.* New York: Vintage/Random House.

Spelman, E. V. (1997). *Fruits of sorrow: Framing our attention to suffering.* Boston: Beacon Press.

Star, J. (1982, May). When every second counts. *Chicago,* 182–187.

Steeves, R. H. (1992). Patients who have undergone bone marrow transplantation: Their quest for meaning. *Oncology Nursing Forum, 19,* 899–905.

Steeves, R. H., & Kahn, D. L. (1987). Experience of meaning in suffering. *Image, 19,* 114–116.

Steeves, R. H., & Kahn, D. L. (1995). A hermeneutical human science for nursing. In A. Omery, C. E. Kasper, & G. G. Page (Eds.), *In search of nursing science* (pp. 175–193). Thousand Oaks, CA: Sage.

Steeves, R. H., Kahn, D. L., & Benoliel, J. Q. (1990). Nurses' interpretation of the suffering of their patients. *Western Journal of Nursing Research 12,* 715–731.

Stein, H. F. (1985). The culture of the patient as a red herring in clinical decision making: A case study. *Medical Anthropology Quarterly, 17,* 2–5.

Stein, H. F. (1990). *American medicine as culture.* Boulder, CO: Westview.

Stein, H. F. (1995). Metaphors of power and the power of metaphor in American biomedicine: A tale of voice, voicelessness, and giving voice. *High Plains Applied Anthropologist, 2,* 131–143.

Stevens, P. E. (1989). A critical social reconceptualization of environment in nursing: Implications for methodology. *Advances in Nursing Science, 11,* 56–68.

Stokols, D. (1975). Toward a psychological theory of alienation. *Psychological Review, 82,* 26–44.

Stouffer, S. A. (1949). *The American soldier: Combat and its aftermath* (Vol. 2.). Princeton, NJ: Princeton University Press.

Street, A. F. (1992). *Inside nursing: A critical ethnography of clinical nursing practice.* Albany: State University of New York Press.

Swanson, K. M. (1991). Empirical development of a middle range theory of caring. *Nursing Research, 40,* 161–166.

Taylor, F. W. (1911). *The principles of scientific management.* New York: Harper.

Tedlock, B. (2000). Ethnography and ethnographic representation. In N. K. Denzin & Y. S. Lincoln (Eds.), *Handbook of qualitative research* (2nd ed., pp. 455–486). Thousand Oaks, CA: Sage.

Tisdale, S. (1986). Swept away by technology. *American Journal of Nursing, 86,* 429–430.

Tomlinson, B. (1999). Intensification and the discourse of decline: A rhetoric of medical anthropology. *Medical Anthropology Quarterly, 13,* 7–31.

Turner, B. S. (1984). *The body and society: Explorations in social theory.* Oxford, England: Basil Blackwell.

van Manen, M. (1990). *Researching lived experience: Human science for an action sensitive pedagogy.* London, Ontario: State University of New York Press.

Warner, J. H. (1997). From specificity to universalism in medical therapeutics: Transformation in the 19th-century United States. In J. W. Leavitt & R. L. Numbers (Eds.), *Sickness and health in America: Readings in the history of medicine and public health* (pp. 87–101). Madison: University of Wisconsin Press.

Warry, W. (1992). The eleventh thesis: Applied anthropology as praxis. *Human Organization, 51,* 55–163.

Watson, J. (1985). *Nursing: Human science and human care, a theory of nursing.* Norwalk, CT: Appleton-Century-Crofts.

Weibel-Orlando, J. (1989). Hooked on healing: Anthropologists, alcohol and intervention. *Human Organization, 48,* 148–155.

West, C. (1993). *Race—Matters.* Boston: Beacon Press.

White, J. H. (1991). Feminism, eating, and mental health. *Advances in Nursing Science, 13,* 68–80.

Wolszon, L. R. (1998). Women's body image theory and research: A hermeneutic critique. *American Behavioral Scientist, 41,* 542–557.

Woods, N. F., Laffrey, S., Duffy, M., Lentz, M. J., Mitchell, E. S., Taylor, D., et al. (1988). Being health: Women's images. *Advances in Nursing Science, 11,* 36–46.

Young, A. (1997). Suffering and the origins of traumatic memory. In A. Kleinman, V. Das, & M. Lock (Eds.), *Social suffering* (pp. 245–260). Berkeley: University of California Press.

Younger, J. B. (1995). The alienation of the sufferer. *Advances in Nursing Science, 17,* 53–72.

Zalumas, J. (1995). *Caring in crisis: An oral history of critical care nursing.* Philadelphia: University of Pennsylvania Press.

3

Living a Life-Sustained-by-Medical-Technology

Dialysis Is Killing *Me*

Rebecca S. Sloan

Renal failure is unique among the end stage diseases in that a mechanical device, the dialysis machine, can perform the functions of the failed kidney. Once a universally fatal condition, death may be held in abeyance by medical technology. Modern advances in technology continue to enhance survival for persons with end stage renal disease (ESRD) as measured by medical outcomes of increased survival time and statistical analysis of numerous quality-of-life instruments (Milde, Hart, & Fearing, 1996; Molzahn, Northcott, & Dossetor, 1997; Sloan et al., 1998; and Wicks, Milstead, Hathaway, & Cetingok, 1997). Interestingly, at the same time ESRD patients' physical and laboratory parameters indicated they were doing well on dialysis, many patients described themselves as very ill or having decreased quality of life.

In-depth interviews with 70 participants (56 ESRD patients and 14 family members) were conducted as they described their experiences of ESRD and its treatment. Using interpretive phenomenology as the philosophical background, their stories were interpreted for common practices and shared meanings of living with ESRD and its treatment. All described concerns of the meaning and significance of holding death in suspension, described as living a life-sustained-by-medical-technology.

At the same time health professions celebrate medical successes, those patients and their families who did not perceive themselves to be doing well cannot be considered inevitable or overlooked. ESRD pa-

118

tients described how dialysis had saved their lives, yet they felt as though they were dying. Patients described this experience as dialysis "is killing *me.*" They perceived that they were no longer who they used to be, could not do the things they used to do, and no longer felt in control of themselves or their futures. Many knew their lives would never be normal again. Some participants described being resigned to this situation, and others were thankful knowing their lives had been spared. Some patients actively sought organ transplantation as a way of regaining normalcy and, thus, them*selves,* while others felt the price of dialysis was too great to pay for the quality of life they endured. This study also explored the experiences of family members of ESRD patients whose loved ones were changed in many ways by the disease and its treatment.

Dialysis therapy is lifesaving for persons who face certain death from ESRD. As good as it is, dialysis therapy does not provide for a normal life. Understanding the ordinary experiences (common illness narratives) of living a life-sustained-by-medical-technology raises questions for healthcare providers assisting ESRD patients and their families, such as: "How prepared are patients for how difficult this treatment will be for them?", "How is hope kept alive for patients beginning dialysis while they are introduced to the difficulties they will encounter?", "Is no treatment better for some people, and who really makes that decision (patients, families, or healthcare professionals)?", and "How are the practices and language surrounding dialysis therapy experienced as oppression for persons who are living a life-sustained-by-medical-technology?" Common illness narratives proffer healthcare professionals the chance to see something that stands in the forefront but is often so familiar it is invisible. For example, frequently healthcare providers rolled out the "poster child" examples of how the therapies for ESRD and compliance to the accompanying medical regimen demands allowed basketball stars to continue to play, persons to dialyze while touring the United States in their Winnebago travel trailers, individuals to resume their careers, or people who have survived 30 years on dialysis treatment—knowing that these exceptions were exactly what made them poster children. Do patients hear the other side of the coin, the Faustian bargain with dialysis technology?

Does this mean healthcare professionals should remove dialysis from the armament against ESRD? Absolutely not. Yet, understanding the meanings created in illness shown in these illness narratives raises new questions for healthcare professionals to ponder. Indeed, the scholarship of this chapter frequently takes the form of questioning the often unanswerable issues that nonetheless deserve thoughtful attention, particularly in the modern techno-medical epoch. This study identified a pattern of living a life-sustained-by-medical-technology unique to the techno-medical epoch. Within this pattern, the theme of "dialysis is killing *me*" illuminated the oppressive healthcare practices to overcome that contributed to this experience.

Advances in Healthcare: Life-Sustaining Medical Technologies

With 283,000 persons currently diagnosed with ESRD, and nearly 40,000 new patients initiated into dialysis therapy every year (U.S. Renal Data Systems [USRDS], 1998), advances in ESRD technology are crucial. However, the dialysis machine was not the objective treatment vehicle patients, families, and healthcare providers expected. It was an integral participant in the experience of living a life-sustained-by-medical-technology. Although the medical outcomes of dialysis therapy are *measured* and *evaluated* through morbidity and survival statistics, morbidity and survival were not statistical measurements to patients and their families. To them, morbidity and survival statistics were *experiences*, integral parts of the bargain struck to sustain life.

Because of its complex technology, the need for continual treatment, and life-sustaining capabilities, dialysis affords a place to study modern techno-medicine and lives-sustained-by-medical-technology. Dialysis is a complex of meaningful experiences

in which one's continued survival depends upon sophisticated technology. . . . Thrice weekly the patients must submit their beings to the "machine"—that magnificent, terrifying, beloved, despised mass of metal, wires and plastic, which is capable of either preserving life or taking a life, which can support daily activities or hinder physical functioning, which may open the door to a productive future or close that same door on a formerly bright career. (O'Brien, 1983, p. 1)

O'Brien's insights reflected the worthiness of understanding ESRD beyond studies of medical outcomes and structured quality-of-life questionnaires. Interpretive scholarship increases understanding of the meaning of living a life-sustained-by-medical-technology that joins human experience and technology in ways that are only beginning to be explored.

ESRD treatment has moved beyond the technology of the artificial kidney machine and now includes organ transplantation. However, organs are scarce, and most individuals seeking a transplant will not receive one. Indeed, only 8,479 transplants were performed for 36,036 persons waiting for kidneys in the United States annually (USRDS, 1999). Those who receive a kidney transplant are given a reprieve from the dialysis machine but are still challenged by invasive surgical procedures, noxious medications, and significant lifestyle changes. In addition to hemodialysis with the kidney machine, other forms of dialysis are available for some ESRD patients. For instance, continuous ambulatory peritoneal dialysis (CAPD) requires up to four or more intra-peritoneal fluid exchanges daily but does not require attachment to a dialysis machine. Other patients meet their dialysis needs while attached to a special machine that performs overnight dialysis treatments. This new, slow intensive home hemodialysis (SIHD) treatment option calls for 6- to 8-hour nocturnal treatments from 5 to 7 nights a week (Cacho et al., 2000). The participants in this study described how traditional hemodialysis was always present for patients and their families. With such an intensive treatment as SIHD, one has to wonder in what ways do treatment regimens ask patients to cross the lines between dialyzing to live and living to dialyze? How does techno-medicine breech the tenets of daily living and become a "strange bedfellow" to the intimacies of family life?

Accompanying a Loved One Sustained-on-Medical-Technology

The toll of ESRD extended beyond the patients themselves. Family members described how their lives were forever changed, too. In a healthcare environment where the *patient* has the disease, the effect of end stage illness on families is given little attention. Frequently families only benefited from services when they could be taught to become more competent home carers. Yet families journey alongside patients in the experience of illness. For many, their concerns seemed invisible to healthcare providers at a time when they were experiencing "intense emotional suffering as they witness[ed] the physical pain and vulnerability of their loved ones" (Cooper & Powell, 1998, p. 63). Little is known about how families accompany a loved one who survives only because of advanced medical technology.

These illness narratives showed how families also endured and suffered as they experienced ESRD and were themselves in need of care. Unlike other serious illnesses, such as cancer and Alzheimer's Disease (Ferrell, Rhiner, Cohen, & Grant, 1991; Mace & Rabins, 1981; K. Parsons, 1997), only a few studies have been conducted to explore the experiences and healthcare needs of family members of ESRD patients (Chowanec & Binik, 1989; Molumphy & Sporakowski, 1984; Rittman, Northsea, Hausauer, Green, & Swanson, 1993; Sloan, 1996; Soskolne & De-Nour, 1989).

Yet, the voices of family members are intertwined in the illness experiences. For example, Bellows described a family facing cancer in a young mother. On the first visit to an oncology specialist, the husband "pulled out family photos and showed them to [the doctor], saying 'I want you to know you're treating the whole family, not just Laura'" (Bellows, 2000, p. G4). Whether Laura lived or died was linked to the outcome of her treatment. Whether their family survived intact was also directly linked to her treatment, and the family made its stake in "their" treatment and need for care known to the healthcare provider.

From a systems theory perspective, chronic illness in one member of the family affects all the members of the family (Bertalanffy, 1968). ESRD patients and families all share in the ramifications of this condition (MacDonald, 1995; Molumphy & Sporakowski, 1984; Wicks et al., 1997), particularly with the accompanying changes in family and workplace roles. These stories or illness narratives remind healthcare professionals how important families are to positive outcomes for ESRD patients and how little research is available on families who accompany a loved one sustained-by-medical-technology.

Loss of the Familiar, Embodied Self: Interpretive Phenomenological Perspectives

In this study, ESRD patients and families commonly described how physical death was a real and anticipated part of the end stage illness experience. Frank (1991) described his experience with cancer, often an end stage illness:

All I could see were the faces I would never grow old with—my daughter, [my wife], my parents. I believed I was going to die, much sooner than later. The pain of my death was in losing my future with those others. My reasons for living have never been clearer. (p. 37)

Though death and loss are very real, patients and families were not prepared for "loss" through the profound changes in personhood experienced by the ill person.

In the literature, conceptualizations of personhood are described using reductionist perspectives resulting in structural/functional (T. Parsons, 1968), cognitive (e.g., Descartes; Dreyfus, 1992), psychological (Erikson, 1959), and social behavioral (Mead, 1962) frameworks. Adding to these helpful reductionist approaches, interpretive researchers have proffered a different, ontological perspective of the self as personhood. Charmaz (1983, 1995) explored the experience of chronic illness from a qualitative perspective concluding "loss of self" was an outcome of continued threat to the integrity of the physical, emotional, and social self. Loss of self was identified by Nochi (1998) in persons who had experienced traumatic brain injuries. In this work using a grounded theory approach, Nochi found that individuals with traumatic brain injury constantly struggled to hold onto them*selves* as others labeled them "abnormal," "wacko," "powerless," or "child-like" individuals. Nochi's participants described how their damaged selves were minimized by professionals who routinely cared for individuals with more extensive injury. As a result of even these "mild" injuries, profound changes occurred for brain-injured individuals and how they saw themselves. They suffered additionally when professionals dismissed the meanings and significances of this experience.

In this study, personhood is viewed from an interpretive phenomenological perspective. Interpretive phenomenology allows exploration of personhood from the perspective of "what it means to *be* a person and how the world is intelligible to us at all" (Leonard, 1994, p. 45). Using the interpretive phenomenology of Heidegger (1926/1962, pp. 234–236), Leonard described persons as having a world that is "constituted and constitutive of the self" (p. 47). Modern Western emphasis on autonomy emphasizes individual power over what happens; Heidegger asserted human beings have only limited ability to alter their lives substantively. Human beings are already situated in worlds by being *thrown* into a particular social, cultural, and historical time by the happenstances beginning with birth. To be human is also to know with certainty that death is the ultimate possibility (Heidegger, 1924/1992; 1926/1962). All human possibilities are in this way finite. Being-toward-death is the most common experience of humans. ESRD is a constant reminder to patients and their families of always being-toward-death. They are thrown into living a life-sustained-by-medical-technology—a life not of their choosing, a life where the ultimate possibility of death shows up as very near.

In interpretive phenomenology, the person is "a being for whom things have significance and value" (Leonard, 1994, p. 49). Because persons experience their worlds on an everyday basis (Heidegger, 1926/ 1962) *things matter,* and the meaning of things can change or hold different meanings for different persons (Dreyfus, 1987). In this study, how the thing called "dialysis" matters was explored not as an object but as an experience. To healthcare professionals in a busy nephrology center, a dialysis treatment is a thing, a technical event that may represent 1 of 90 or more vascular access connections, uneventful treatments or dialysis runs, and machine clean-up procedures done daily—only to be repeated tomorrow. To the patient, a dialysis treatment is some*thing* different than what dialysis personnel do for them. As dialysis patients must "submit their beings to the machine" (O'Brien, 1983, p. 1), it is also an experience with great meanings that, of course, cannot be separated from the chrome-plated efficiency of medical technology.

From a phenomenological perspective, personhood is more than a personality attribute or psychological label. Phenomenologically, personhood is explored in its full essence—that is, what it means to be a person in a particular situation at a particular time (Leonard, 1994). This study focused on what it meant to be a person who has experienced life-sustained-by-medical-technology, a person who has experienced dialysis is killing *me,* and what this critical illness meant to their family. As Frank described, "critical illness leaves no aspect of life untouched . . . your relationships, your work, your sense of what life is and ought to be—these all change, and the change is terrifying" (1991, p. 6).

Methods

Through interpretive phenomenology, this research aimed to elucidate understanding of: (a) living a life of chronic illness, (b) living a life-sustained-by-medical-technology, (c) the meaning of that experience for patients and their family members, (d) how these experiences were made visible or invisible by the social practices and relationships that surround healthcare, and (e) how oppressive healthcare practices could be improved to provide better care to patients and their families. Interpretive phenomenology led to scholarship that pursued thinking as being on the way of a twisted wood-path (Heidegger, 1967/1998, p. xiii), where thought may either lead down a blind alley or to a clearing of understanding. With the goal of providing better care to patients and their families, each illness narrative in the study contributed to this scholarship in two ways: (a) narratives opened up a particular area of questioning, and (b) narratives became part of a larger data set contributing to a journey of scholarship exploring what it meant to be a person who lives a life-sustained-by-medical-technology where the questions to be asked are not yet clear. Although each study is complete, the path of scholarship is never ending. There was a continual back and forth as thinking pursued new possibilities of understanding illness and its treatment as experienced by patients and their families.

The lasting element of thinking is the way. And ways of thinking hold within them that mysterious quality where thought moves forward and backward, and that indeed only the way back will lead thinking forward (Heidegger, 1959/1982). Understandings about living a life-sustained-by medical-technology came from repeated hermeneutical analyses of all of the narratives shared by persons with ESRD. Only recently introduced to nursing research, "Heidegger recast hermeneutics from being based on the interpretation of historical consciousness to revealing the temporality of self-understandings" (Diekelmann & Ironside, 1998, p. 243). This way of thinking was further informed by 20 years of nephrology nursing practice. Personal experience as the daughter of an ESRD patient contributed to this work as well.

Participants

The 56 ESRD patient participants included both male and female dialysis or kidney transplant patients who had once been on dialysis therapy. The 14 family member participants included husbands, wives, adult children, siblings, and in-law relatives of ESRD patients. Participants were from 28 to 94 years of age and, thus, provided data across a wide

range of individual and family developmental stages. This diversity contributed to the study findings. Institutional review board approval was
obtained from each of the participating study sites prior to initiation of
the studies.

The study participants were recruited from two large university-
based outpatient dialysis centers, one in the Midwest and one in the
Midsouth. The dialysis population in the Midwest setting was 73% African American, 24% Caucasian; 51% male and 49% female. ESRD was
the result of diabetes (31%), hypertension (34%), glomerulonephritis
(13%), and other causes (19%). In the Midsouth setting, the dialysis
population was 31% African American and 59% Caucasian; 54% male
and 46% female. Diabetes, hypertension, and glomerulonephritis were
the most frequent causes of ESRD in this population as well. In this
study, 11 participants came from the Midwest site and 59 came from
the Midsouth site. Participants had to be at least 18 years of age, non-
institutionalized, and able to provide informed consent.

As the researcher worked in the Midsouth facility as a research
nurse, she was familiar to many of the patient participants but did not
have direct patient care responsibilities for any of the participants. Dialysis patients and their family members clinically known to the researcher
were invited to participate. Initial approaches to patients and family
members were made in person. Later in the studies, nephrology nurses,
physicians, social workers, or previous participants also introduced potential participants following snowball enrollment techniques.

In an effort to gain trust, remove potential perceived power differen-
tials between the researcher and the participants, and to increase comfort with the project, patient–family member dyads were encouraged
to select the time and place of the interview. They also chose whether
they were more comfortable being interviewed separately or together.
Some participants elected to be interviewed as dyads and some elected
separate interview times. At times a patient or family member was interviewed without completing the interview with the other, usually due to
schedule conflicts or when changes in the health of the patient refocused
the energies of the patient and family. This also happened when either
a patient or family member "had a story to tell," but the other was more
reticent. Sometimes it was the absence of a family member that was the
story—and the patient needed to share that as well (Sloan & Rice,

2000). This approach allowed for multiple types of illness narratives to be heard including: (a) the patient's story, (b) the family member's story, or (c) their story together. Each approach brought useful insight into the common experiences of living a life-sustained-by-medical-technology; yet each offered different perspectives as well.

Interestingly, all of the study participants chose to be interviewed before or after the patient's scheduled dialysis treatment or a clinic appointment. They elected to be interviewed in a quiet area within each of the two study sites rather than in their homes or other settings, saying they spent so much time in these facilities they felt "at home" in these settings. Interview space was found in either comfortable conference rooms or in a private area equipped with casual chairs.

Gathering Narrative Data

Just as there is no single method for conducting interpretive phenomenological scholarship, there is no single set of criteria used to assure integrity of the research findings. Yet, to not make clear what efforts were made to do so would fail to reflect the scholarliness of interpretive research. In her personal program of study, the researcher holds closely to the following: bringing forth the voices of the participants, not her own; holding herself open to new thinking through presenting interpretations to other scholars, rather than confirming her own preunderstandings; challenging her thinking by reading broadly in other professional disciplines and the humanities in search of shared meanings; and finally, opening up unrecognized meanings and practices that would "reveal, enhance, or extend understandings of the human situation in the world" (Diekelmann & Ironside, 1998, p. 244). The method for this study and the researcher's efforts to provide integrity to this process follow.

After informed consent was obtained, nonstructured interviews lasting from 1 to 2 hours were conducted with persons with first-hand knowledge of living everyday with ESRD. This approach allowed participants to guide the direction of the interview content, choosing which experiences to share rather than limiting discussion to a predetermined set of questions about their lived experiences with ESRD. The following questions were useful in beginning the interviews: "How did you come to know you (or your loved one) would have to start dialysis?" and "What

did dialysis mean to you when you first started dialysis and what does
it mean now?" Finally, they were asked to reflect on what they thought
was ahead of them and how they described their future of possibilities.

The questions included in each interview varied following the lead
of the participants and the stories they wanted to tell. Clarifying information was gathered using questions such as: "Describe a time when
this happened," "Give me a for instance," or "Please tell me a story that
says it all about what it means to be a dialysis patient (or family member)." Soon recognizable recurring experiences (themes) were identified, and specific questions were asked about those shared events or
things. This was not done to validate the findings but to challenge and
elucidate an emerging common experience that had multifaceted ways
of showing.

The Hermeneutic Circle: Helical Interpretations

Healthcare providers can understand the experiences of living a life-
sustained-by-medical technology even "though we do not all experience
or live in the same worlds, these worlds can be described, talked about,
and discovered" (Benner, 1994, p. 116). Benner described how this is
possible based on the "three-fold structure of understanding" or fore-
structure (p. 71). Diekelmann and Ironside (1998) described this framework to include our background practices (fore-having), which provide
familiarity with our world and serve as the perspective for interpretation
of phenomena (fore-sight). According to these authors, preunderstandings (fore-conceptions) "describe our anticipated sense of what our interpreting will reveal" (p. 243). Baker, Norton, Young, and Ward (1998)
described how Heideggerian hermeneutic researchers

assume that human communities share an understanding of their lived experiences that is shaped by culture, language and other social practices. This is not
simply to imply that all persons hold the same understandings, but to indicate
that understandings are shaped by experiences in particular worlds. (p. 549)

So it is in the world of patients and families living with ESRD.

From a Heideggerian perspective, human beings are always already
in the world as interpreters of experience. In this research, the hermeneutical process moved within a circular structure that was also helical
(though never linear), complete, yet never ending. Each additional nar-

rative brought new understandings that were added to what was always already understood by the researcher. Thus, looking across an accumulating collection or ensemble of narratives gathered to date contributed to an ongoing inquiry. In Heideggerian hermeneutics, the process was described as circular:

> Just as the interpretive researcher moves back and forth between the parts and the whole of the text, the stance of the interpreter must shift from understanding and imaginatively dwelling in the world of the participant to distancing and questioning the participant's world as other. The interpretive researcher engages in cycles of understanding, interpretation, and critique. (Benner, 1994, p. 116)

The analysis was also helical in that initial questions evolved into more sophisticated understandings after some time, even years later, yet the researcher was able to go back to the original thinking and questioning in a continuous, yet never identical, pathway of thinking. Describing the analysis process as "moments" will demonstrate how this is possible for hermeneutical interpretations to be both circular and helical. The three different moments in the overall research process reflected the helical nature of interpretation:

Moment 1. "In the moment" interpretations occurred simultaneously with gathering the original narrative
Moment 2. Interpretations of each individual narrative as an entity to itself
Moment 3. Interpretations of an ensemble of narratives collected across a life's work (to date) of inquiry

These three moments of helical activity were not linear but occurred as a never-ending interplay, going back and forth as one moment informed the next and came back to the original questioning. As Diekelmann and Ironside (1998) described, hermeneutics "has no beginning or end that can be concretely defined but is a *continuing* experience for all who participate" (p. 243). Using this approach, understandings were affirmed by additional narratives, previous understandings were expanded by new facets and new questions, or previous understandings were critiqued, overcome, and rethought completely. With narratives being collected across an extended period of time, the researcher was simultaneously engaged in analysis activities that were responsive, reflective, and interpretive. A detailed description of each moment follows.

First Moment: "In the Moment" Interpretations

Interpretation was an ongoing process that both preceded and began at the moment the interview was occurring. As humans do, the researcher brought preunderstandings and anticipations to the interviews, yet remained open to new interpretations and understandings of others. By initiating analysis as the words were being said (which is what humans do in understanding our personal worlds in our daily lives), the researcher responded to what was heard, asked more questions, and clarified thoughts with the participants even as those thoughts were forming. Thus, clarification of what individuals said or meant occurred during the interview itself, holding open opportunity to again contact individual participants for clarification as the transcripts were being analyzed. The researcher and the participants both shaped and were shaped by the interview experience. After each interview field notes of thought and observations were written for future reference.

Second Moment: Interpretation of Individual Narratives

Individual narratives were audiotaped at the time of the interview, transcribed verbatim, and rechecked against the original tape recordings for accuracy. Punctuation was corrected so as not to alter the meaning of the spoken narratives when put into textual form. Additional data, often obtained from field notes, such as observations of body language, facial expressions, and eye contact were added to the typed narratives to bring the reader as much information as possible from the original interview. All identifying information was replaced with pseudonyms. The tapes were kept in a secured area with a locked cabinet.

Analysis of individual transcripts was initiated immediately after data collection. During this process, each transcript was read multiple times. In interpretive phenomenological scholarship, a theme is a common recurring experience or concern, and a pattern represents the highest level of interpretation and is "present in all the interviews, and expresses the relationships of the themes" (Diekelmann & Ironside, 1998, p. 244). Stories or portions of texts of the illness narratives that resonated with common experiences and common meanings were identified. Each narrative was given numerous descriptive codes to assist in identifying the common experiences (themes) as revealed by the individual participants. Patterns also were named as they emerged. A computer-based data management software designed specifically for use with qualitative research, Atlas.ti (Muhr, 1997), assisted in data management of the study. With nearly 4,000 pages of narrative collected to date, retrieving specific stories or important passages in order to read across texts was impossible without a software program. Atlas.ti does not analyze the data but provides a word-processing format for organizing, identifying, and retrieving this information.

Third Moment: Interpretation of an Ensemble of Narratives Across an Emerging Inquiry of Scholarship

In the third moment, the individual transcripts were re-viewed as an *ensemble of narratives* formed from all of the narratives contained in an ongoing, ever-growing exploration of a phenomenon (in this case, living a life-sustained-by-medical-technology). Here the ensemble of narratives was read as a whole multiple times, and the literature was searched again. In this third moment, common themes and patterns described by ESRD patients and family members were identified and analyzed and their common meanings described. Themes were affirmed, combined, challenged, altered, or eliminated through reading across the ensemble of narratives. Dialogues with the literature were written to reveal unwarranted interpretations.

To keep open the possibility of alternative interpretations, the transcripts and interpretations were consistently and regularly offered for critique by others. These individuals included participants, as well as nonparticipant ESRD patients and families to determine if understandings were credible. The counsel of experienced nephrology nurses, physicians, and social workers was sought to read interpretations and final research reports. Indiana University School of Nursing has formed a "hermeneutic circle" of scholars who support each other's programs of research. This community of interpretive researchers meets regularly and assisted with narrative analysis and interpretation development. Since 1992, the researcher's scholarship and thinking have benefited from participation in the University of Wisconsin–Madison Advanced Nursing Institute for Heideggerian Hermeneutical Studies. This interdisciplinary community of interpretive scholars meets annually to engage in dialogue that turns on what is ownmost to the philosophical thinking that is the grounding of interpretive research. Through these avenues, the researcher has direct access to the individual and collective support of a community of experienced researchers who graciously shared their time and effort to assure the integrity of interpretive research. However, it is the readers of the research who are the final arbitrators of the integrity of the research findings.

Interpretive phenomenology brings new understandings of a phenomenon by opening up the complexity of what seems simple and everyday. Though interpretive research is not intended to be predictive or generalizable, the findings do have to be useful. Three hundred thousand persons undergo dialysis treatment every day in the United States. This study opened up what it meant to live a life-sustained-by-medical-technology as revealed by the bargaining practices associated with an agreement with technology and the loss of the familiar, embodied self. Ever more technologies are being used to sustain individuals with other "end stage" diseases. How useful these findings will be to understanding those phenomena is yet to be known. Only the readers of this work—patients, families, and professionals—will be able to answer that question.

Living a Life-Sustained-By-Medical-Technology

The pattern of living a life-sustained-by-medical-technology was present in every narrative in the study. The theme of dialysis is killing *me,* a shared meaning of living a life-sustained-by-medical-technology, was identified to some degree in each of the narratives as well. The theme of dialysis is killing *me* was described from various perspectives in these illness narratives as a loss of the familiar, embodied self. Patients were challenged by the duality of a therapy that offered survival, perhaps at the cost of "living," yet not to enter into this agreement meant imminent death. These illness narratives described how it was that this impasse was overcome. ESRD patients and families described the meaning of living a life-sustained-by-medical-technology and provided new ways of thinking for healthcare providers to improve care to these individuals.

Yet, at the same time dialysis was revealed as "killing me," it was also revealed as "saving my life"—an interesting paradox of living a life-sustained-by-medical-technology. Many ESRD patients seemingly adjusted to the demands of dialysis, and their lives were "saved" to carry on active and engaged lives. Others were not so fortunate. For them, survival occurred but "living" was elusive. From these stories came a new understanding of what it meant when patients felt dialysis is killing *me.* These were also the stories persons facing dialysis may not hear.

What would it mean to patients and families to hear these stories of both sides of the coin as they consider this bargain they are about to enter? Perhaps hearing how dialysis "kills" at the same time it "saves" would allow individuals to make more informed choices. Is it possible providing both sides of the coin would assist patients and their families to anticipate and participate in these decisions with a greater degree of understanding? Maybe hearing the stories of other patients would assist them to adapt as they find their own way in this unfamiliar world. Would hearing the stories of the bargaining practices of patients on life-sustaining high technology therapies help them to find meaning for themselves in this pact with technology?

Dialysis Is Killing Me

Although all dialysis patients experienced changes in their lives necessitated by their illness and its treatment, some ESRD patients found their very existences at risk. Such was the story told by Kurt and Carol, a Caucasian couple, 50 and 34 years of age, respectively. Coming from a poor, rural area of the Midsouth, neither Kurt nor his wife had ever heard the word *dialysis* before Kurt's illness. Though Kurt hated his dialysis treatments from the beginning, he said, "I had to. Either that or die." Thus Kurt entered into an agreement with the dialysis machine hoping that his life would be saved. He did not know how profoundly his life would be changed. Kurt's story told how without treatment for his renal failure, he would surely have died. Yet Kurt found that the life-saving treatments were also "killing me," causing him to actively seek organ transplantation. He described how he came to know this was his only chance to live:

K: I wanted a kidney [transplant]. I just wanted to live longer, I guess.
R: But obviously you wanted to live without having dialysis.
K: Right. Right. I couldn't live long on that dialysis machine I know that now. I couldn't do it. I just couldn't do it.

Kurt's physical condition on dialysis was stable, and his laboratory parameters were within expected limits, but he perceived that he "couldn't live long on that dialysis machine":

R: I don't understand.
K: That machine kills me. That machine kills me every day. I just don't want to go through it [dialysis] again.

R: Uh huh. Is it physically painful?

K: No. It's just the idea of going down there and getting stuck every day. . . . It's just in your mind I guess. . . . The days I felt good, it was still on my mind, I gotta go back in the morning, you know. It was always in my mind, you know, where I gotta go in the morning. . . . It was on my mind for three years.

R: Is it mentally or is it emotionally? Was it the dread? Can you describe it?

K: I just knew it. I just knew it.

Kurt described the meaning to him of living a life-sustained-by-medical-technology. He offered not that *dialysis* was killing me, but that dialysis was killing *me*. His description reflected a common meaning of patients experiencing loss of the familiar, embodied self. This loss was as acutely felt as a physical loss. Dialysis interrupted familiar ways of being-in-the-world, as does any illness. Yet the language of "killing" was strong and full of violence. Clearly the personal experience of dialysis was not one of resting peacefully in a recliner chair as one received treatment.

Carol was soft-spoken and somewhat overwhelmed by the changes in their lives brought about by Kurt's ESRD. She told more about how the loss of the familiar, embodied self that Kurt had experienced affected her life, too:

If you live with somebody that's on dialysis (long pause). That's rough. You know, the things they go through, the way they act, and they go through just terrible depression. Or he did. He was real bad. Sometimes they get to where they don't want to live. . . . He would always tell us that we just didn't know what it was like. You know it's terrible watching them get stuck with needles. . . . And he was always just down, and of course dialysis made him deadly sick. He just more or less stayed in the house, laying down, because he had nausea or trouble with his blood pressure.

A life-sustained-by-dialysis was not asymptomatic and continually brought the loss of the familiar, embodied self to the forefront of one's existence. Kurt's personhood was becoming intolerable for him and unfamiliar to his family. He knew he "could not live long on that machine" and found a way to preserve his personhood through seeking kidney transplantation. The average waiting time for a cadaver kidney is 2 years; Kurt remained on dialysis for 3 years waiting for a kidney to become available. Now no longer tied to dialysis therapy, Kurt described what his new kidney meant to him:

It was rough the first month or so. But I'm glad I went through it. It was rough. But it was worth it. [Not] going to that machine. Well, I love it. I just hope that I never have to go back [to dialysis]. I feel good all the time.

Earl, a 30-year-old Caucasian man, elected to try CAPD treatment for his ESRD. He chose CAPD because the technology of hemodialysis "drives me crazy." Although CAPD is less technical, Earl still felt the unrelenting intrusion of ESRD and its treatment on his life. This was so pervasive that he described losing his familiar, embodied self to the extent of obliterating his familiar identity entirely:

People don't really understand how bad it is I don't think. . . . 'Cause it's a constant 24-hour battle all the time. Workin' this catheter, tryin' to keep the exit site clean. . . . It's a 24-hour deal. I mean it's really around the clock. But you know, here I am—"Kidney Disease Man."

Although some might interpret Earl's comment as a use of humor or bravado, another possibility is that Earl's perspective had shifted from having the disease to being the disease. Once a person, then a "person with kidney disease," Earl described a loss of his familiar, embodied self. Now he was left with only the kidney disease. In Earl's eyes, his personhood was reduced to a cartoon caricature of the healthy person he once was. He said, "I wouldn't even know what it feels like to be normal. I mean I really wouldn't." He saw transplantation as a way out of his present circumstances—a way of getting him*self* back. When asked what he expected after transplantation, he said:

Who knows? Maybe I'll feel like a new person. I think I probably will. I'll tell you one thing I'd really like to know is how damn bad do I really feel? I mean I feel like I feel pretty bad. I hope I get to test it and see. I just don't do anything outside in the sun. I've had some trouble sleeping. I was taking iron pills. I mean, that was something that was really affecting my rest, too. I can't even rest good at night because things [blood chemistry levels] were so out of whack. I'm jittery. I'm nervous. I can't sleep. I wouldn't wish this [dialysis] on anyone. Wouldn't wanna see anyone go through it. The reason I wanted to stay away from hemo[dialysis] is because I've seen all the needles and people down there and you know? I mean can it be that good for you? People pulling your blood out? I mean I guess it helps. It's good. But I just don't like the thought of that. It drives me crazy.

Stories like those from Kurt and Earl raised many questions. How do healthcare providers prepare and accompany patients and families as they make treatment decisions and navigate the challenges of those treatments? Are there better ways to inform and help patients and their families anticipate and cope with losses related to the habitual body? How can patients be assisted to find new everydayness and familiarity, if not comfort, in their new embodiments?

Kurt's family provided some insight into practices that preserved personhood and influenced their experiences in the dialysis unit. Paradoxically, it was not *what* the dialysis nurses did but *how* it was done that made all the difference to Kurt and his "feeling cared for," safeguarded, and recognizable for his uniqueness and personhood:

K: I love them nurses—all of them. It's just like family. You see them every other day for three years. Well, they're family really.
R: You sensed that they cared for you?
K: Well, I know they did. It was just the way they treated me. They tried to be good to me. Well, they treat you good. If I wanted anything I'd ask them, and they'd come over there and check me.

Kurt's story went well beyond the dialysis unit and was a lesson for how healthcare providers did support the familiar, embodied selves of persons regardless of their particular health problems. Patients expected their healthcare providers to be technically competent. But it was when healthcare providers engaged in behaviors that made patients feel safe, looked after, and cared for that patients' personhoods were preserved, acknowledged, supported, and valued. These behaviors must be timely and responsive. Kurt loved "them nurses," just like family. What is embedded here is that although nurses may monitor machines for frequent and rapid physiological changes, the nurse-as-family checks on *me*.

Precarious Patients/Precarious Families

Carol also described a threat to their financial security since Kurt was unable to be the family breadwinner. When Kurt could no longer work, their small savings were quickly depleted. He applied for Social Security disability, but it would be months before any money was received. Carol had never worked outside the home and now she had to support the family from tips made waiting tables at the local diner. Although some of his huge medical expenses were covered by insurance, the rest of the family did not qualify for assistance with their living expenses or family medical bills: "Like *he's* on Medicare, but we don't qualify for a medical card or anything like that. We don't qualify for anything like that. It just kind of makes it hard. And you worry a lot."

Few individuals had sufficient sick leave to keep a paycheck coming in more than a few weeks. Disability benefits took months to process before any monies reached the family. Bills kept coming in the mail. Antonio, a 70-year-old Caucasian male, had this experience in paying for treatment of his ESRD: "It just floored me when I saw the bills. I've got stacks of bills [indicates 2 feet]. I can't make sense of them. Well, it's a worry." Although financial worries that were part of their bargain with technology created stress, participants told how their ability to provide for their families, their usual way of being in the world, had been forever compromised. No longer persons in control of their lives, they were persons dependent on others.

Narratives from individuals with ESRD and their family members revealed previously concealed common meanings of living a life-sustained-by-medical-technology for those who encounter ESRD and its treatment every day. The stories described how current entitlement programs influence the preservation of personhood in ways that were never intended. How is it that research in ESRD focuses on improving medical technology, yet ignores the financial threats that accompany new technologies for dialysis patients and their families?

Teddy, a 57-year-old African American man, still had a family to raise when he was diagnosed with ESRD. After 30 years of working for the same company, he was too ill to keep his job. He asked for help from the United Way and the Veterans Administration, but both denied his request. He spoke of how damaging this experience was to his personhood when he said, "I worked for 30 years. It's hard to ask somebody to help you" (Sloan & Rice, 2000, p. 11). A proud, honest, religious man, Teddy found himself in an impossible situation. To overcome this impasse, he had to become a liar before any help was offered to him:

T: And that's sad when they make you lie to get help. And they do make you do that. To get help, you got to lie. And that's hard for some people.
R: Especially if you've spent your life being an honest person.

T: If you want to be (honest). You can't do that and run through that
system. You can't do that. You have to change. And tell them what they
want to hear in order for them to help you. And that's sad. . . . And
when you go down there and ask them to help you, and then they say
"Well, you make too much money"—and you're not even working you
are so sick! . . . "Well, you make too much money 'cause your wife
works." They made me wait almost six months before they gave SSI
[Social Security Insurance] to me. It took every penny I had to wait
until they started my SSI. They ought to make it work so if you're
disabled, you ought to get better help than you do. There ought to be a
helping hand out there for you. 'Cause it's nothing that you wanted to
do [get sick]. It's something that just happened. (Sloan & Rice, 2000,
p. 12)

Like Teddy, Milt was too ill to work, and no paycheck was coming
in for his family. With four children to feed, Milt tried desperately to
get food stamps while he was waiting for his disability to be approved.
"I wanted to get food stamps for me and my kids. They told me to get
out of there" (Sloan & Rice, 2000, p. 12). These stories described how
the dialysis patient and family continued to need food and clothing and
to meet rent or mortgage payments. In addition to the usual healthcare
needs of families, the crisis of the patient's ESRD resulted in stress-
related illness in other family members, particularly the patient's carer.
In today's economy, many employers offer no insurance to their employ-
ees, or offer insurance that is unaffordable. Programs that allow individuals to continue medical coverage through a previous employer (e.g.,
COBRA) can cost upwards of $400 a month. Kurt's family soon faced
moving in with relatives just to get by. Strauss (1975) described the
financial drain facing the ESRD patient:

The point at which it becomes clear to the patient that his survival depends,
henceforth, on hemodialysis—is usually the moment of financial truth . . . he
has entered into partnership with a machine. Above all, the machine is a greedy
and inexorable consumer of time and money (p. 111).

In time, the majority of Kurt's medical expenses would fall under
Medicare reimbursement. What will never be covered are the costs to
Kurt's personhood in order to survive the financial burden of living with
ESRD.

Terms of the Bargain: Making a Deal for Time

As difficult as it was to live a life-sustained-by-medical-technology, many dialysis patients did manage to continue dialysis for many years. Not all patients described dialysis as killing; some thought it was saving their lives. As Elonzo said, "God bless the dialysis machine" (Sloan, 1999, p. 504). Even those individuals, though, told of the hardships that accompanied living a life-sustained-by-medical-technology. DeShaundra, a 33-year-old African American woman, described how dialysis had saved her life but also how the very core of her personhood became unfamiliar to her:

D: I only did it because I had to. Because it kept me alive.

R: What was it about dialysis that was so bad?

D: Because it made me feel like I was dying. It's not that I felt physically bad, and I had my good days and I had my bad days. But it's just the act of doing the dialysis that just (long pause) . . . it just made me feel like I was dying. 'Cause it wasn't me, you know? I'm the type of person that was, like, on the go constantly. And dialysis ruled my life now.

For DeShaundra, rather than regaining her life, she felt her life was appropriated by dialysis, "it's like my life revolved around dialysis." However, as a young mother, she desperately wanted to be alive for her family. The family not only sustained her but provided avenues for her to be a wife and mother, preserving her personhood. Stories like DeShaundra's revealed that families gained time through this bargain with technology. Similarly, Regina, a 30-year-old African American woman, was accompanied to the interview by her husband, Benjamin. Their three preschool children played about their feet throughout the interview. She, too, described that she was willing to pay the price of living, saying, "whatever it takes," she wanted to "be with her family."

Carl, a 66-year-old African American man, described how an unexpected child came into his life when his son and girlfriend put their new baby up for adoption. At his age, Carl had decided against dialysis, saying, "I just said I was going to go on and die" (Sloan, 1996, p. 156). Dialysis made it possible for Carl and his wife, LaVonia, to accept this child into their own home to raise. Even though his everyday life would now include needles and nausea, he was willing to pay this cost for time to raise this child.

Not only were families with young children willing to do "whatever it takes" to be there for them, families at the other end of the life span entered dialysis for the same reasons. Andy, a 70-year-old Caucasian man, said he only initiated dialysis treatment so that he could continue to care for his terminally ill wife. He exclaimed, "That dialysis! Where it'll keep you alive, it don't do much for your livin'." These profound words revealed the chasm that existed between "surviving" and "living." Even so, dialysis does make survival possible.

Participants described why surviving, even if not "living," was so important to them. Facing death from ESRD himself, Andy also knew that his wife's chemotherapy had failed. He initiated dialysis because he had promised his wife he would be there to care for her. After his transplant, he was well enough to care for his wife for a year before she died: "The only thing I've got time for is takin' care of my wife. She's got terminal cancer. . . . I've got more stamina now. I can hang in there longer, much longer." Andy described how "dialysis is saving my life" even while he recognized "it don't do much for your livin'." It appeared that "family" is a key element in understanding the bargaining practices that occurred for individuals living a life-sustained-by-medical-technology. Practices that influenced the preservation of personhood were as simple as "being there" to parent a child or care for a loved one. As Carl said, "After I got that baby, I went on dialysis . . . and I could take care of that baby right. So she's five years old now (Carl's eyes sparkle). Me and her's real close. . . . She saved my life" (Sloan, 1996, p. 157). As outside viewers of Carl's experience, healthcare providers might assume that modern medical technology is responsible for Carl's survival. Carl, however, credits the baby with his decision to enter an agreement with dialysis technology, saying he took the baby in and now sees that "life is too precious to die" (Sloan, 1996, p. 158). These stories reveal how family served both as a factor affecting the bargaining process and a means of preserving personhood.

Although some families grew in strength from the challenges of living a life-sustained-by-medical-technology, other families could not bear it. Roger, a 36-year-old Caucasian man, told how "the biggest thing for me was losing my family." After many years of caring for Roger, his wife "just couldn't take it anymore" (Sloan & Rice, 2000 p. 13).

Not all families help patients with ESRD survive. Sometimes, the participants developed "family ties" with other dialysis patients. Asa explained, "and you have a dialysis family, because you spend 3 hours a day, 3 days a week with the same people." Dolores spoke of how close she became to the families of other dialysis patients over the endless hours spent in waiting rooms: "You get to know those people. And they get to know about you." Sometimes the new "family" comprised the dialysis personnel. As Kenny said, "those two gals who came up there to run the dialysis machine just made me feel like I was home or something. They were more like my daughters [than nurses]."

Stories of breakdown were also heard describing healthcare providers who had little interest in patients as persons. Donna, the 44-year-old sister of a dialysis patient, recalled conversations with her brother, Alex:

Something he said was whenever someone dies, he always says the nurses don't care. They'll have somebody else in that chair next time. It just leaves an empty chair for another one. I think that's always bothered him that your life can be gone and the people you spend 3 days a week with don't show any emotion or don't really care. There'll be somebody else in the chair next time.

With 40,000 new patients initiating dialysis every year, empty spaces in dialysis units do fill very quickly. Although patients had some understanding that someone was "in that dialysis spot" before them, they also experienced a significant threat to personhood when those who provided care for them appeared not to care when a death occurred. How is it that healthcare providers coped with the inevitability of their ESRD patients dying with behaviors that are interpreted as depersonalizing? This story calls for healthcare providers to examine how care is given that preserves personhood for ESRD patients and families.

When the Price of Survival Becomes Too High

In the above story, Carl's contract with medical technology continued to be worth attendant losses related to his familiar, embodied self. Andy's story ended differently. Six months after his wife's death, which was the reason Andy said he needed to survive, he died from complications from immunosuppressive therapy. One has to wonder if he reached a place where the reason he entered this pact with high-tech therapy was no longer worth the bargain.

Pain also contributed to loss of the familiar, embodied self. Sometimes the pain was so overwhelming, patients withdrew from dialysis. Rosita, a 39-year-old African American woman, received a renal transplant 5 months prior to the interview. She described how her physical pain on dialysis contributed to depression and emotional despair so profound she wanted to die. More than a physical and emotional manifestation, she also experienced a threat to her personhood. Prior to her illness, she had fulfilled the roles of wife and mother. Now she saw her*self* as a burden to her family. Her sense of self was so diminished, she wanted to end her life:

I never will forget I was in so much pain. And I just asked God to take my life. And my husband told me, "Don't you ever let me hear you say that again." And I got to the place where I was so depressed that I thought I was a burden on him. And I told him I didn't want to be a burden to him. And he told me [tears in her eyes], "You are my wife. You know that's what I'm here for."

Yet, "pain gives of its healing power where we least expect it" (Heidegger, 1971, p. 7). Rosita shared how even when she was in pain, she was empowered by her husband's love and support. She told how she regained enough strength to seek another way out of this impasse through kidney transplant. Most patients are informed of the option of organ transplantation at the time they initiate dialysis treatment, or earlier in their illness trajectory if possible. Unfortunately, this often occurs at the same time that disease, worry, and pain bring patients to their knees. Once patients reject the notion of organ transplant, they may not be asked again to consider this option (Sloan, 1996). Now the burden of seeking transplant falls to the patient. Patients have to be strong enough to ask (often repeatedly) for the transplant team to meet with them. They must pass numerous and extensive physical, laboratory, and psychological tests to determine their eligibility. They must be strong enough to ask a family member to consider donation and wait through the donor's eligibility testing. If no family member is willing to donate, or if no family member matches the patient, then the patient must be strong enough to wait months or years for a cadaver organ to be available, all the while undergoing a treatment that is killing *me*. Because of her family's support and love, Rosita mustered a resoluteness that sustained her, and she found the strength to seek organ transplantation. She vowed, "If this kidney rejected, I would have another. If the other one rejected, I would do anything to keep from going on dialysis. Because that's not a life. It's not."

As healthcare providers come to a new understanding of dialysis is killing *me,* new questions arise regarding how personhood is influenced by this procedure. How are healthcare professionals to know when the terms of the bargain are exhausted for an individual and family, and treatment is too costly? How do healthcare professionals justify being accomplices to procedures that challenge the line of "do no harm"— procedures that patients describe paradoxically as killing them at the same time their lives are saved? Is this not a place of restless to and fro? How can healthcare providers better accompany and assist patients who feel dialysis is killing *me?* Perhaps out of the experiences of peril comes the knowledge needed to escape or overcome the dangers of entering the pact between human being and machine. The stories also revealed practices to draw upon to overcome the impasse of this pact. Sometimes, participants told stories of overcoming one impasse only to have that replaced by another.

From One Impasse to Another

As the above stories revealed, patients and families encountered one impasse after another: agreeing to life-saving treatments that resulted in dialysis is killing *me,* making choices to pay overdue medical bills while trying to make a week's medications stretch to cover a month, having to beg or lie for financial support or not be able to feed their families, or waiting months or years on the transplant waiting list while they endured treatments that robbed them of their familiar, embodied selves. Organ transplantation was another treatment option, but it was not available to everyone. Patients had to be healthy enough to meet eligibility requirements, strong enough to navigate the eligibility process and wait months or longer for an organ, and lucky enough that a match would be found. Others described the impasse where this option was not available to them at all and they had no choice but to continue dialysis. Sometimes this was due to a significant co-existing physical condition, such as obesity or heart disease; sometimes patients described a financial barrier.

Nathaniel, a 37-year-old Caucasian man, received a kidney transplant 10 months before the interview. He became paraplegic at 18 years of age after surviving a terrible accident. Nathaniel made an excellent recovery, restoring an everydayness with his new habitual body as a paraplegic. Several years later, a new threat to this now familiar, embodied self manifested when he developed ESRD from poor bladder management. He described how he could not survive long on dialysis, even though his laboratory and physical findings indicated he was doing well:

I just thought it [dialysis] was a death sentence. I mean, you'll never live through it. You know? I mean, you can survive. But see, the dialysis machine doesn't know the difference between good and bad in your body. It just sucks everything out. The good iron, the calcium. All the things you need goes right out, too . . . I think a lot of people have (given up hope). You get used to seeing people come, and all of a sudden you don't see them anymore. You say, "Now where's what's her name?" "Oh, she died last week." And I thought, "I'm going to die real soon." Because like from week to week I could see my face drawing up. I was losing so much weight I looked like I was going to die any minute. I was getting so little. Real little. I thought I was going to die, too.

In Nathaniel's case, his physicians expected him to lose weight as his body adjusted to a new weight without edema. Mineral and electrolyte changes were part of the expected outcome of dialysis therapy. Once faced with the impasse of dying from renal failure or accepting a life-sustained-by-medical-technology, Nathaniel now found himself at a new impasse. On the one hand, he spoke of dialysis keeping him alive but also how that life was one of unrelenting restrictions and demands:

It don't ever leave you. It don't ever leave you. You've always got it. It's always there. Like every time you go to eat, you can't have that. Potato chips, sorry. Bananas, sorry. Anything you like, sorry. But we got some tasteless crackers here you can have. So every waking minute of your life, you are thinking about it.

Finding dialysis to be an impossible situation to "live" with, Nathaniel desired a kidney transplant. His desire for an organ transplant brought him to another impasse. Nathaniel had been told that he was not a candidate for transplantation:

I was on dialysis like that, oh, for a good long time. I can't remember exactly how long. It seemed like a year or close to it. And then I asked them, "Hey, you know, I want a transplant." Now this was back before I was married. All I had was Medicare, and it don't cover your prescription costs. So they said, "Well, Nathaniel, you're just not a candidate." I thought, "Well, being in a wheelchair, I could understand." But it turned out it wasn't the wheelchair at all. I don't have the money to buy my medicine. They were thinking for me, because that's more money than I make, what my medicines costs—and without no insurance . . . (long pause).

In Nathaniel's story "it wasn't the wheelchair at all." He understood that access to organ transplantation, the medical treatment of choice for ESRD (Franklin, 1994), was denied to him for financial reasons. Whether this was the true situation or not is unknowable. At this time, persons are not denied access to therapy for ESRD merely for financial reasons, although persons were once denied because of age and now may be restricted if their weight is not within certain guidelines (Pagenkemper, 1999). At the time of Nathaniel's initiation into dialysis therapy, there were restrictions on how long transplant medications would be reimbursed by federal funds. Perhaps this was where this perception originated. Or perhaps the healthcare professionals thought his long-term health would not be enhanced by the stresses of surgery and continual immunosuppressive therapy. Whatever the "truth," Nathaniel believed the decision was made for monetary reasons—reasons he was helpless to change.

Nathaniel told how his dialysis nurse arranged for him to meet her sister, a wonderful woman whom Nathaniel married a few months later. He described a sudden change in his transplant eligibility and said sarcastically, "It was just miraculous! After I got married all of a sudden I *was* a candidate for a transplant. It turns out she works for a hospital. Got real good insurance. So that's what the deal is." Once facing a lifetime of dialysis treatment with no other options, Nathaniel now had the means to escape dialysis through the miracles of organ transplantation. Through a chance meeting, a love affair, and a "real good insurance" policy, Nathaniel received a kidney transplant and new hope for the future. He said, "It already seems like it was 20 years ago, and it [the transplant] was only in September. Seems like I never had the kidney disease now." Even though Nathaniel had renewed hope and no longer just survived on dialysis, but lived with a kidney transplant, living a life-sustained-by-medical-technology was difficult. He found that he had entered a new bargain with technology, that of organ transplantation. Although many persons, sick or healthy, struggle with difficult children, unhappy marriages, and mountains of unpaid bills, Nathaniel found his life choices limited, as he also had to "protect" his new kidney as well:

N: I love my wife, but now it's just about to the point where I'm just about ready to leave her because my stepson is driving me crazy. But I can't (long pause) . . . because she has insurance. So, it's either lose your kidney or you stay where you are miserable. So, I'm kind of in a Catch-22 situation.

R: Your choices are gone because of this?

N: Yeah. I have to stay with them. And I love her to death, I really do. . . . I've been debating getting a job and stuff. And I'm scared to do that too, because I don't know what holds my future [sic]. And I've been on disability 18 years now. I've got my Social Security going and things like that. Oh, I'd hate to mess that up! But I turned down some good jobs. But what happens if I get a pressure sore or something and I can't go to work? And they say, "Well, Nathaniel we gotta have somebody fill your spot." And then what about Medicare? Can I get it back? . . . And I've had people to call me, collecting from Lakeside hospital. She says, "Can you send $30 a month?" I say, "Yeah, but I might not be able to fill my prescriptions."

Nearly one-fourth of transplants are lost within 3 years due to graft failure, infection, or inadequate immunosuppressive therapy (USRDS, 1997, p. 107). It is unknown how many of those transplant failures are due to patients trying to "stretch my medications to the end of the month." Cyclosporine, a potent anti-rejection agent, costs hundreds of dollars a month and is only one of the many medications ESRD patients are prescribed for organ transplantation and their underlying medical conditions. Some participants described how they sometimes entered drug research projects to assure a supply of medication. As Carol described, "Thank goodness that they started this study again because at least for another year we're not gonna have to worry about getting cyclosporine." Sonny, a 29-year-old Caucasian man, told how he worried constantly that he would not be able to buy his immunosuppressive medications, "'Cause that's the main thing for me—the cyclosporine." Sonny knew that without anti-rejection medication, the "gift of life" would be lost.

Nathaniel's personhood as a "transplantable patient" was colored by his healthcare providers' view of his tenuous financial picture. Initially, Nathaniel perceived that his carers were "thinking of me" when they recognized that he did not have sufficient financial or insurance support to maintain the expensive medication therapy that accompanied organ transplant. In the end, even with "a good insurance policy," he had to juggle paying one medical expense and not paying another. For many participants, their choices were caught between purchasing much needed medication, paying for rent, or feeding the family. These are stories of facing one impasse after another as part of entering the Faustian bargain. Although "stealing from Peter to pay Paul" is not uncommon in any of our lives, the stake for ESRD patients was survival itself. Organ transplantation was indeed a gift of life, but it was a "hungry" gift that required constant and expensive feeding. The price of the bargain was higher than patients anticipated.

Nathaniel's story revealed how the treatment of ESRD encompassed much more than the successful application of knowledge to provide technology to sustain life. Nathaniel perceived a loss of him*self* as long as he remained on dialysis, experienced as a loss of the familiar life touchstones of who he was, that his future of possibilities was limited, and that he was at an impasse in his ability to change this course. Even after a kidney transplant, he lived in fear that he would lose this gift of life if he could not maintain the unrelenting financial burden. Pharmaceutical companies do offer indigent programs to help individuals meet their medication needs. However, each company only supports their own drugs (and sometimes only selected medications). Applications have to be filled out, processed, and approved; medications have to be sent and dispensed. Weeks can go by. Most programs only provide medication for short periods of time, 1 to 4 weeks, and then the process must begin again. Although patients are relieved and grateful when these medications arrive, they are immediately concerned about their next month's medication supply. Nephrology social workers spend huge amounts of time facilitating the paperwork of indigent drug applications for ESRD patients; although these activities are on behalf of ESRD patients, they actually draw social workers away from patients directly. While the nation struggles with the best expenditure of our healthcare dollars, has society addressed how the various entitlement programs may cost more in administrative and clerical support than the relief provided? Further, what does it "cost" an ESRD patient's personhood to have to ask for help over and over again? What are the experiences that result in the surrender of an individual's touchstones of personhood when seeking benefit from medical entitlement programs?

Exploring "Breakdown" to Reveal Successful Ways of Preserving Personhood

Bringing the Invisible Into View

Sometimes the preservation of personhood became apparent through the experiences of breakdown, those times that further diminished personhood. Patients described how they received satisfactory physical care and expected their healthcare providers to be competent but felt a loss in being cared for. For these patients, their lived experience of dialysis resulted in a loss so complete that they experienced a personhood of invisibility (Sloan, Junod, Potter, & Ventrello, 1999). Families were made to feel invisible as well. Donna's family was made to feel worthless and invisible by the hospital staff caring for her brother:

That first night we came [to the hospital] it was in the night. [Midnight] or so, and we were just going to sleep in the lobby. The lobbies are not made to accommodate very many people. Everything was full. Even floor space. And so we went down to the main lobby and just laid down. My aunt and my uncle were in their 60s, you know, and they laid down across the couches. And a security guard came at 5:00 in the morning. Which is 4:00 our time. And made us get up! And made us put our feet on the floor because they were going to unlock the [hospital] doors. And they made us get up! And we had only been layin' down about 3 hours whenever they came and had us get up. And he just come and started beating on the back of the couches! And said, "Put your feet on the floor! Sit up! Sit up! Put your feet on the floor!" . . . It wasn't like we were camped out there for the duration. I mean, we got a motel room for the next night. But at that time of the night! And Alex wanted us to be there close.

In this story, the hospital security guard objectified Donna's family and failed to see them as people in a particular context—a family in crisis. The family was not at the hospital in the middle of the night because they chose to be. They were exhausted, had no information on Alex's medical situation, and were doing the best they could to be there for him. Donna's family perceived that their plight was invisible to the hospital security guard, someone who allegedly spent much of his time around persons in just these sorts of circumstances.

Not only did Donna perceive that the needs of her family were invisible to those who should have understanding, she recognized the threat to Alex when he was treated like an inanimate object by his healthcare providers in the dialysis unit: "They were just in and out. Just like you were just another block of wood layin' there and you know, it was like you never had feelings. . . . Nobody ever told you anything."

Alex told of loss of his familiar, embodied self as his situation went unrecognized by those caring for him:

I don't think the people really know what you go through, you know? The nurses expect a lot out of you, "you should do this" or "you should do that." But they don't really realize how emotionally rough that is as far as mentally a strain on you.

This is a story of breakdown, where those who were needed to care became blunted and insensitive to their patients. A lack of understanding of what patients were experiencing was manifested in the care being given. For example, healthcare providers often chastised dialysis patients for eating too much salt or drinking too much water and failed to respond to the efforts the patient *was* making. Although healthcare providers recognize the health risks of these behaviors, how do these illness narratives uncover these meanings that add to understanding the whole story of ESRD? Carers want to facilitate self-care behaviors that contribute to positive outcomes for patients. One of the hallmarks of psychology is that all behavior has meaning. Understanding the meanings behind all behaviors, positive and negative, brings new possibilities for improving outcomes and experiences of those who face ESRD. This story also reveals how little is known about how patients and their families hear what health providers say.

What is meaningful to patients and families and how these meanings are shaped by the caring practices and the delivery and monitoring of these extreme treatments needs further exploration. For example, Keith, a 69-year-old African American man, frequently was chastised for his "excessive" water intake. For Keith, however, perpetual thirst was a common everyday occurrence of dialysis therapy compounded by his diabetic condition: "See I'm a diabetic. And maybe, if you were a diabetic . . . you're going to crave water. Because it has a burning inside you" (Sloan, 1996, p. 109). Keith faced an impossible situation of trying to meet the demands of one disease and its treatment while a second condition with conflicting needs was also present. How often do healthcare providers criticize patients for failing to meet our expectations in diet and medication compliance without understanding what the meanings of those demands have for patients? Although water restriction is a medical necessity, what does it *mean* to live for months or years without end thirsty and craving water?

Not only did healthcare providers evaluate patient compliance to diet and medication, providers also evaluated patients' compliance with expectations for self-care or rehabilitation. Participants described how healthcare providers referred to them as noncompliant, passive, or unmotivated to help themselves. Particularly singled out were individuals who slept through their dialysis treatments rather than being active and engaged participants in self-care. Do healthcare providers understand that "being motivated" does not always assure that positive patient outcomes occur? For example, Tyrone initiated dialysis treatment while finishing graduate school. He described how his peers and healthcare providers thought he had a wonderful opportunity to study while undergoing hours of dialysis therapy. Though a motivated student, Tyrone found that he could not focus long enough to finish a crossword puzzle, let alone study for chemistry exams, at the same time his body and brain were experiencing rapid homeostasis changes resulting from dialysis treatment. These stories call healthcare providers to new thinking about how important it is to understand the life story or the personhood of the patient in order to accompany those faced with invasive, demanding, and relentless ESRD treatment modalities.

Stories of breakdown also revealed positive ways ("Concernful Practices," Diekelmann, 2001) that overcame threats of objectification and depersonalization. Alex and Donna also described a nurse they would never forget:

D: Her name was Kristi. I remember that because she came over and said "Mr. Arensman, where are you from?" And he said, "Smoketown, Illinois." When you say that, nobody knows where Smoketown is. She said, "Well, that's where my mother's from." Come to find out we knew her family.

A: She took care of me all that day. She came up to my room twice. Then when I was moved upstairs and checked on me and talked to me for awhile.

D: And before you left, she brought you a little cup that said State University, like a little pottery thing. Something for him to bring home from there.

This was not a story about the gift of a pottery cup. It was a story about the welcoming and gathering, knowing, and connecting practices of a nurse (Diekelmann, 2001; Diekelmann & Diekelmann, 2000, 2001) The story reflected the small acts, gifts of time, and caring that preserved personhood. Surrounded by high-tech machines and frightening procedures, this nurse demonstrated welcoming practices that forever shaped this family's experience. These concernful practices overcame depersonalization and made patients feel valued, "at home," and "safe." A smile, a chat, a moment to accompany another facing perilous times reflect the "splendor of the simple" (Heidegger, 1971, p. 7). In today's healthcare settings, providers lament how they have no time to spend with their patients, talking to them, touching them, "being with" them. From all indications, these small acts will decrease as the push for reducing healthcare costs through shorter hospital stays, healthcare staff reductions, and focus on "billable" services continues to determine the amount of time providers can spend with patients and families. The decreased time providers spend with patients makes it difficult to attend to the personal attention and small acts that can overcome the objectifying and depersonalizing experiences for patients and their families.

Hearing the Language of End Stage *Disease and Preservation of Personhood*

As participants described the loss of the familiar, embodied self, sometimes they encountered minor, but irritating, disruptions in their personhoods and lifestyles. Other times, the intrusion of ESRD and its treatment resulted in substantial alterations in the familiar, embodied selves to the point where they felt totally depersonalized and invisible. The language of ESRD contributed to this depersonalization. For patients with ESRD, death, the ultimate threat to personhood, was very near. Not only was death always in the forefront, it was also experienced through the very name applied to this condition—*end stage* renal disease, suggesting an imminent and inevitable death.

Walter was interviewed 6 months after a cadaver kidney transplantation. He describes discovering he was labeled as *end stage*. The emotional strain of knowing that he was facing a terminal condition with very limited options is recounted:

They had on my papers ESRD, you know? And then when I finally found out what it stood for, that it was just the fact that they're callin' it the "end stage" renal disease. This is the end of it right here. There ain't nothing else, you know? It's more than you can't drink somethin' today or can't eat somethin' today. It's not tomorrow either. . . . And when you're in your last . . . it's just the last thing, you're in your last stage. You're ready to leave that stage, you got to go either (long pause) go on with God or you're either gonna get a transplant or somethin'. . . . But when you get kidney disease and go on dialysis, it's just—that's just it.

In interpretive phenomenology, the future exists as possibilities. Walter's story evoked what it means to carry this label, clearly aware of the experience of being-toward-death. For Walter the label *end stage* represented a closing down of his future. It was one more threat to his being, who he was, his personhood. Medicine and healthcare require a specialized language; however, rarely is this average everyday language explored for how it shapes patients' experiences. To a patient, end stage means death, the end, "there ain't nothing else" coming. For healthcare providers, end stage renal disease can mean other things: (a) It is a diagnostic category for describing nonrecoverable renal failure, and (b) it qualifies persons for federal medical care reimbursement. To understand language as experienced, that is from the perspective of those who carry this label, healthcare providers have to be open and seek out the stories of patients and their families. Is it time to eliminate medical language that, however useful, oppresses and closes down patients' future of possibilities? Has the term *end stage* reached its culmination and utility and is now a label that oppresses?

This study calls for rethinking the language of ESRD and exploring new labels. Social worlds are constituted by the symbols of language that permeate communication and interaction. Yerby, Buerkel-Rothfuss, and Bochner (1995) described how:

People live in a social world created or sustained through their communication. . . . Symbolic meanings are unique constructions—that is meanings change from culture to culture and from situation to situation. . . . The generation of meaning is a symbolic and socially constructed activity in the sense that individuals react to events and to each other on the basis of what the behavior represents in their social world. (p. 7)

Thus, end stage means something different as experienced within the world of patients than it does within the world of providers. What language would patients use to describe this stage of their disease? Is this a place for developing with patients and their families a neoteric health-care language for ESRD?

Walter experienced depersonalization and objectification not just from the language of ESRD. He was further labeled a "bad patient." His familiar day-to-day life was often diminished by noncaring behaviors of his healthcare providers who criticized his efforts to meet the physical goals of therapy that required constant restriction in his food choices. He was labeled a bad patient because he was unable to control all of his laboratory parameters and behaviors to his healthcare providers' sat-isfaction. Although he perceived himself as trying very hard to comply, his healthcare providers labeled him as "noncompliant," challenging his personal attempts at self-control, self-determination, and-self worth:

Well, my BUN [blood urea nitrogen—a laboratory value that indicates kidney function] run about 60 when I was on the machine. And like I said, the phospho-rus was the only thing. And when they brought the labs around, instead of saying you done good on this or you done good on that and tried to give you some encouragement, they'd say, "Your phosphorus is up again. You're gonna have to do better than that." Just chew you out on what didn't look good. They never said what you did good on. And sometimes when you're on dialysis, be-cause you know that's an everyday struggle. Every morning when you get up, you got the same thing to look forward to when you go to bed at night. Then you get up the next morning, you know, you got the same thing to look forward to as you did the day before. The same struggles, the same troubles and every-thing. And instead of them trying to give you a word of encouragement, or trying to give you something to look forward to when you go back over there, all you were gonna get was chewed out.

These illness narratives resonated with many accounts of how op-pressive labels shaped persons' experiences on life-sustaining technolo-gies. This study does not find that these are intentional outcomes of healthcare. Perhaps in an urgency to provide quality care and correct or eliminate patients' physical problems, healthcare providers forget the meanings and significance of their verbal exchanges with patients. Does being pressed to care for many patients in a short period of time encour-age healthcare providers to overemphasize the negative and neglect or fail to appreciate the meaning of this approach to patient? This study fills out the story of techno-medicine and adds knowledge about the meanings and significances of the common experiences (including lan-guage) of ESRD patients and their families.

Techno-Medicine and Healthcare: Forgetting the Whole Story

No one questions that the dialysis machine has prolonged the lives of countless individuals. The work of medical scientists who seek ever more efficient and effective technology is important work. However, this study showed that the interface between person and machine is a complex phenomenon about which healthcare providers know very little. This study does not find dialysis machines to be evil nor that healthcare providers are intentionally indifferent to their patients' well-being. Yet, these stories revealed that life-prolonging dialysis treatment can be described as "killing *me*" and that carers can fail to take into account the whole story of living a life-sustained-by-medical-technology.

For Heidegger, the claim of "techno-scienticism" included the forgetting that there is more to the advent of meaning and significance than reductionist methodologies choose to address (Heidegger, 1926/1962; Heidegger, 1938/1999). The practices of science have meaning and significance beyond the reductive methodologies employed. For example, in the practice of medical science individual human beings can be reduced to the point that statistical manipulations of projected outcomes limit medical treatment options (e.g., those overweight are frequently ineligible for organ transplantation, and the "care map" determines whether patients are responding appropriately to prespecified indicators of their illness and treatments) (Heidegger, 1926/1962). When humans are reduced to problems, objectifying human experience can occur:

> If we make a problem of "life," *and then just occasionally* have regard for death *too, our view is too short-sighted.* The object we have taken as our theme is *artificially and dogmatically curtailed* if "in the first instance" we strict ourselves to a "theoretical subject," in order that we may then round it out "on the practical side" by taking on an "ethic." (Heidegger, 1926/1962, pp. 363–364)

When death is viewed within the practice of science as a biological event, the story is simple and straightforward. Without maintaining biological integrity, there can be no survival and, thus, no living. Thus, maintaining life at the biological level becomes the overarching raison d'être to the healthcare system. Yet, this story is also inadequate since, as this story revealed, death can be experienced while there is still biological life. Treatment for some of these ESRD patients was experienced as death-inducing or "killing *me.*" It is the experiences of being-toward-death that matters not just biological death itself. In techno-medicine and healthcare, science as an approach forgets it is not the whole story. Interpretive phenomenological scholarship, through describing the *common meanings* of living a life-sustained-by-medical-technologies reveals, extends, and challenges the necessarily incomplete techno-medical story. Thus, science cannot apprehend the whole and, thereby, dismisses the rest of the story.

In a scientific view, meanings are considered "unprovable," and merely "subjective and personal" (Grondin, 2000). Though meanings can be quantified, this approach is always incomplete. For example, in psychology, when meanings are measured as attributes, though generalizable, they become the ultimate reductive view because they ignore context and history. Meanings that are situated, contextual, and historical are never captured in the story of techno-medicine. Yet, the demands of providing healthcare necessitate that providers extend their understandings to include as much of the whole story as is ever possible. This is the contribution of interpretive scholarship to contemporary techno-healthcare.

Modern technology is neither good nor evil in and of itself. Rather, what matters is how human beings have been driven to embrace technology. This is the claim technology makes on humans. Technology is both: (a) a "human activity" and (b) "means to an end":

The two definitions of technology [as human activity and as means to an end] belong together. For to posit ends and procure and utilize the means to them is a human activity. The manufacture and utilization of equipment, tools, and machines, the manufactured and used things themselves, and the needs and ends that they serve, all belong to what technology is. (Heidegger, 1954/1977, pp. 4–5)

In this study human activity is required in development and manufacture of the dialysis machine and is part of the technological picture, the envisioned "end" of sustaining life through the "manufacture" of cleansed blood through removal of life-threatening toxins. Lives are saved and attempts to improve the quality of life are made. In this endeavor, though, scientists strive to meet these goals by limiting their attention to physics, anatomy, pathophysiology, and how the dialysis machine can be improved to better meet the physiologic needs of ESRD patients.

Scientists engage in a never-ending quest to advance current technologies and to bring forth new ones to meet the needs of those with ESRD. Technology has served humans well as a means to the end of sustaining life for ESRD patients. However, technology's twofold definition (as a human activity and a means to an end) alone does not help healthcare providers understand the meanings of living a life-sustained-by-medical-technology. Does the definition of technology as the application of current medical knowledge in any way inform persons of what it means to enter into a pact between humans and machines?

The dialysis machine is an engineer's dream of mechanical construction, finely tuned passive and active filtration membranes and biochemical exchange media. This death-defying machine of steel is impressive, with complex tubing hookups and Spartan design. It removes waste products effectively and efficiently and can be manipulated by dialysis personnel to achieve the biological goals specified. Yet all the engineering schematics available do not reveal what it means to live alongside this mechanical wonder, to live a life-sustained-by-medical-technology. How is dialysis experienced as a Faustian bargain?

Entering a Faustian Bargain With Techno-Medicine

Living a life-sustained-by-medical-technology reveals the meaning of being appropriated by technology (Heidegger, 1938/1999)—caught between humanity and machine. It is here that life-sustained-by-medical-technology was experienced in ways that patients and families described across a continuum from life-saving dialysis therapy to dialysis is killing *me*.

Dialysis machines were once very scarce. Now, through modern manufacturing techniques and enhanced reimbursement mechanisms, access to the artificial kidney machine is virtually unlimited in the United States. Thus, the "standing reserve" of dialysis equipment has encouraged an environment in which access to dialysis therapy has significantly limited death due to kidney failure alone. This standing reserve of dialysis equipment and personnel has given way to routinization of the dialysis process, with dialysis healthcare professionals finding meaning in how many "runs" are done per day, how quickly dialysis setups are "turned over" from one shift to the next shift, and mathematical measurement of dialysis adequacy. Quality of life is measured in terms of reducing mortality and morbidity on a per annum basis and is evaluated by how closely laboratory values are brought into a "right relationship" by the dialysis treatment. Rarely were patients asked to provide information on their experiences of how they were doing or what it was like to live a life dependent on dialysis or transplant technology.

What does dialysis mean for someone who enters into the world of dialysis only hoping to stave off death? How informed is this decision? Do patients begin dialysis with a commonly held view of a dialysis patient resting quietly reading, writing letters, or doing homework while the treatment is going on? Certainly some of these study participants tolerated dialysis better than others, but none spoke of productive times during the treatments. Even incredibly difficult chemotherapy has an end in view that sustains most cancer patients, but dialysis patients have no end to treatment.

At what point do some patients survive ESRD physically yet experience death of the self and begin saying it is killing *me*? How prepared are patients for this possibility? Are patients routinely prepared or assisted along the way to anticipate a sense of loss, sometimes so extreme the patient or family no longer recognizes the person they once knew? Are patients encouraged to talk with other patients who have found dialysis "life-saving" as well as "killing"? What is known about the commonly held expectations and meanings of beginning dialysis? Once dialysis is initiated in what ways and how often are patients given the opportunity to change their minds? When biological survival is present but patients discover that, for them, this is merely the shell for living, how is care made available to those patients? All of these questions should be researched to increase healthcare providers' understandings and to create a research base from which care is provided to patients.

As observers of their loved ones' struggles and pain, ESRD family members described being powerless. They experienced only that someone they loved and knew was "lost" to them, unrecognizable in the person before them, and they were unable to control or even understand what was occurring. How is it that ESRD patients become "unknown" to the family who holds them dear? As is the case in many chronic illnesses, families described painful experiences in which they could do little to change the disease and could only offer to be a companion along a fearful, exhausting, and uncertain path. Further, they revealed how difficult accompaniment proved to be:

As a daughter, I learned firsthand about the pain that a family experiences when a loved one is diagnosed with end stage renal disease. Pain so intense, so scary, that often we (a "good" family) couldn't bear to enter my father's room. I learned that even words of hope can bring tears—the risk of opening your heart to pain again, knowing hope can evaporate in a heartbeat. (Sloan, 1996, p. 202)

Are the families of patients with ESRD routinely seen as "in need" of healthcare? If the stress and emotional pain of accompanying a loved one with ESRD constitutes needing healthcare support, who attends to the family's needs? Though families may be informed of the physical changes expected with dialysis treatment, how do healthcare providers prepare them for the possible loss of the familiar ways of being of their loved ones? Would knowledge of this potential allow families to prepare for changes or to actively develop ways of preserving personhood within the family structure, rather than being caught by surprise?

Lessons Learned

This study extends the story of living a life-sustained-by-medical technology. However, it is not without limitation. Participants in this study were heavily weighted toward hemodialysis treatment over transplantation (2:1). It is possible that those strong enough to seek a way out of dialysis therapy were also strong enough to recognize their sense of loss and verbalize their experiences. On the other hand, even those who did not articulate a sense of dialysis is killing *me* directly described tremendous losses to them*selves* while surviving end stage renal disease. Perhaps they have passed beyond a stage of being able to do something about this circumstance and are resigned to this situation. An example comes from Elonzo, a 54-year-old African American man, who said, "Like dialysis is the end, and then you die" (Sloan, 1999, p. 505).

Another limitation of this study is that the voices of healthcare providers, doctors, nurses, and technicians are not included. Continuing study of the common meanings of caring for a patient with ESRD would contribute to a more complete story. How do nurses experience assisting patients with ESRD about beginning dialysis or other treatment options, including no treatment? Although healthcare professionals know what to do to withdraw someone from dialysis, how is it to accompany patients and families during the rethinking of treatment decisions throughout the course of treatment? How do the dialectical concerns about providing adequate information for informed consent coexist with the belief in a self-fulfilling prophesy as a result of describing undesirable symptoms or reactions to treatment? Is there any evidence that anticipating the possibility that dialysis may be experienced as killing discourages patients from selecting dialysis and/or encourage poor outcomes? Or does the knowledge that some patients experience dialysis as killing prepare them by providing anticipatory guidance, influencing compliance and positive outcomes?

These illness narratives told how healthcare providers, either through action or language, influenced the preservation or loss of the familiar, embodied self of patients. Unflattering labels routinely used to describe patients, such as "passive," "non-compliant," "too old," or "too fat for transplantation" (Sloan, 1996), further influenced the care that patients received. Perhaps healthcare providers could rethink how language and actions, specifically those that involve control and compliance, are manifested through technology and the manner in which they are used.

Dialysis units are run on schedules reminiscent of major airports—persons arriving and departing from an assigned dialysis chair, with only minutes between "passengers" for technicians and providers to ready equipment for the next treatment. Providers are called on to "turn over" three or more shifts of patients daily, often working 10 to 12 hours per day. Dialysis workers are caring individuals who want their patients to do well. Yet, for each patient in the dialysis unit, there is also a dialysis machine, a machine that has to be prepared with tubings and fluids, cleaned with chemicals, and refitted very quickly for the next patient's treatment, a machine that calls for the health provider's attention with every alarm. Every time the machine "calls" to the dialysis worker, the machine must of necessity come to the forefront, with the patient slipping into the distance. No one intends for patients to feel invisible, yet these stories reveal that they commonly do.

The everydayness of living a life is taken for granted; that is, everyday lives are nearly invisible except at times of breakdown (Dreyfus, 1992; Heidegger 1926/1962). Breakdown, or times when the normalcy of everyday life is disrupted, calls for examination of what, as shown in this study, healthcare providers often take for granted. Thus, when the technology is not providing the expected outcome, providers examine *the technology* to see what is wrong or seek ways to improve the outcome. In ESRD, scientists have spent years "examining the technology" and "improving the outcome." For example, numerous studies have been conducted comparing one dialysis filter with another and one medication against another and monitoring laboratory results. Medical scientists have examined whether waste products in the blood can be removed more efficiently by dialysis machines three times weekly or by continuous ambulatory peritoneal dialysis methods. Bioscientists have ventured into, and conquered for the most part, the unknowns of organ transplantation. Pharmacologists have been very successful in developing tools to help delay the inevitable in this end stage illness. As Nagle (1998) found:

More than ever before, the technologies of healthcare have begun to supplant the human experience of an illness experience. . . . The question remains as to whether the technological imperative of healthcare has shifted the focus of nurses from people to machines. (p .78)

This is not to imply that the presence of this shift is an intentional devaluation of the human experience by providers. Rather it is a reflection of techno-medicine in a for-profit model of delivering healthcare that turns on power as control, order, and predictability. As technology becomes an ever more prominent feature in modern life, it is timely to explore the influence on patients, families, and healthcare providers in living a life-sustained-by-medical-technology. This round dance of humans and machines reveals a Faustian bargain that can rob personhood in return for biological survival. This study not only shows how techno-healthcare forgets the whole picture but also provides new understandings of making a pact with dialysis or kidney transplant. How can illness narratives assist in providing healthcare professionals with more understanding and insights of the whole picture of patients and their families living a life-sustained-by-medical-technologies?

References

Baker, C., Norton, S., Young, P., & Ward, S. (1998) An exploration of methodological pluralism in nursing research. *Research in Nursing and Health, 21,* 545–555.

Bellows, S. (2000, April 13). Fight of her life. *Indianapolis Star,* pp. G1, G4.

Benner, P. (1994). The tradition and skill of interpretive phenomenology in studying health, illness, and caring practices. In P. Benner (Ed.), *Interpretive phenomenol-*

ogy: Embodiment, caring, and ethics in health and illness (pp. 99–128). Thousand Oaks, CA: Sage Publications.

Bertalanffy, L. von. (1968). *General systems theory.* New York: George Braziller.

Cacho, C., Guthrie, B., Priester, A., Murray, E., Newman, L., Blankschaen, S., & Weiss, M. (2000). Slow Intensive Home Hemodialysis (SIHD): The University of Cleveland Experience. *Nephrology News & Issues, 14*(4), 36–41.

Charmaz, K. (1983). Loss of self: A fundamental form of suffering in the chronically ill. *Sociology of Health and Illness, 5*(2), 168–194.

Charmaz, K. (1995). The body, identity, and self: Adapting to impairment. *Sociology Quarterly, 36*(4), 657–680.

Chowanec, G. D., & Binik, Y. M. (1989). End stage renal disease and the marital dyad: An empirical investigation. *Social Science and Medicine, 28*(9), 971–983.

Cooper, M. C., & Powell, E. (1998). Technology and care in a bone marrow transplant unit: Creating and assuaging vulnerability. *Holistic Nursing Practice, 12*(4), 57–68.

Diekelmann, N. L. (2001). Narrative pedagogy: A Heideggerian hermeneutical analysis of lived experience of students, teachers, and clinicians. *Advances in Nursing Science, 23*(3), 53–71.

Diekelmann, N., & Diekelmann, J. (2000). Learning ethics in nursing and genetics: Narrative pedagogy and the grounding of values. *Journal of Pediatric Nursing, 15*(4), 226–231.

Diekelmann, N., & Diekelmann, J. (2001). *Schooling learning teaching: Toward a narrative pedagogy.* Unpublished manuscript.

Diekelmann, N., & Ironside, P. M. (1998). Hermeneutics. In J. Fitzpatrick (Ed.), *Encyclopedia of Nursing Research* (pp. 243–245). New York: Springer Publications.

Dreyfus, H. (1987). Husserl, Heidegger and modern existentialism. In B. Magee (Ed.), *The great philosophers: An introduction to Western philosophy* (pp. 254–277), London: BBC Books.

Dreyfus, H. L. (1992). *What computers still can't do.* Cambridge, MA: The MIT Press.

Erikson, E. (1959). Identify and the life cycle. *Psychological Issues, 1,* 18–64.

Ferrell, B. R., Rhiner, M., Cohen, M. Z., & Grant, M. (1991). Pain as a metaphor for illness. Part I. Impact of cancer pain on family caregivers. *Oncology Nursing Forum 18*(8), 1303–1309.

Frank, A. W. (1991). *At the will of the body: Reflections on illness.* Boston: Houghton Mifflin Co.

Franklin, P. M. (1994). Psychological aspects of kidney transplantation and organ donation. In P. Morris (Ed.), *Kidney transplantation: Principles and practices* (pp. 532–541). Philadelphia: W. B. Saunders Company.

Grondin, J. (2000). Continental or hermeneutical philosophy: The tragedies of understanding in the analytic and continental perspectives. In C. Scott & J. Sallis (Eds.), *Interrogating the tradition: Hermeneutics and the history of philosophy* (pp. 75–83). Albany: State University Press of New York.

Heidegger, M. (1962). *Being and time* (J. Macquarrie & E. Robinson, Trans.). New York: Harper& Row, Publishers. (Original work published 1926)

Heidegger, M. (1971). *Poetry, language, thought* (A. Hofstadter, Trans.). New York: Harper & Row, Publishers, Inc.

Heidegger, M. (1977). *The question concerning technology and other essays* (W. Lovitt, Trans.). New York: Harper Torchbooks. (Original work published 1954)

Heidegger, M. (1982). *On the way to language* (P. D. Hertz, Trans.). New York: Harper & Row. (Original work published 1959)

Heidegger, M. (1992). *The concept of time* (W. McNeill, Trans.). Cambridge, MA: Blackwell Publishers. (Original work published 1924)

Heidegger, M. (1998). Preface. In McNeill, W. (Ed.). *Pathmarks* (pp. xiii). New York: Cambridge University Press. (Original work published 1967)

Heidegger, M. (1999). *Contributions to philosophy (from enowning)* (P. Emad & K. Maly, Trans.). Bloomington: Indiana University Press. (Original work published 1938)

Leonard, V. W. (1994). A Heideggerian phenomenological perspective on the concept of person. In P. Benner (Ed.), *Interpretive phenomenology: Embodiment, caring and ethics in healthcare and illness* (pp. 43–63). Thousand Oaks, CA: Sage Publications.

MacDonald, H. (1995). Chronic renal disease: The mother's experience. *Pediatric Nursing, 21*(6), 503–507.

Mace, N. L., & Rabins, P. V. (1981). *The 36-hour day: A family guide to caring for persons with Alzheimer's disease, related dementing illnesses and memory loss in later life.* Baltimore: The Johns Hopkins University Press.

Mead, G. H. (1962). *Mind, self and society.* Chicago: University of Chicago Press.

Milde, F. K., Hart, L. K., & Fearing, M. O. (1996). Sexuality and fertility concerns of dialysis patients. *American Nephrology Nurses' Association Journal, 23*(3), 307–315.

Molumphy, S. D., & Sporakowski, M. J. (1984). The family stress of hemodialysis. *Family Relations, 33,* 33–39.

Molzahn, A. E., Northcott, H. C., & Dosseter, J. B. (1997). Quality of life of individuals with end stage renal disease: Perceptions of patients, nurses and physicians. *American Nephrology Nurses' Association Journal, 24*(3), 325–333.

Muhr, T. (1997). Atlas.ti (Version 4.1) [Computer software]. Berlin: Scientific Software Development.

Nagle, L. M. (1998). The meaning of technology for people with chronic renal failure. *Holist Nurs Pract, 12*(4), 78–92.

Nochi, M. (1998). Struggling with the labeled self: People with traumatic brain injuries in social settings. *Qualitative Health Research, 8*(5), 665–681.

O'Brien, M. E. (1983). *The courage to survive: The life career of the chronic dialysis patient.* New York: Grune & Stratton.

Pagenkemper, J. J. (1999). Obesity: A serious risk factor in transplantation. *Nephrology News & Issues, 13*(8), 58–62.

Parsons, K. (1997). The male experience of caregiving for a family member with Alzheimer's disease. *Qualitative Health Research, 7*(3), 391–407.

Parsons, T. (1968). *The social self.* New York: Free Press.

Rittman, M., Northsea, C., Hausauer, N., Green, C., & Swanson, L. (1993). Living with renal failure. *American Nephrology Nurses Association Journal, 20*(3), 327–331.

Sloan, R. S. (1996). *A hermeneutical study of the medical treatment decision for end stage renal disease patients and their families.* Unpublished doctoral dissertation, University of Kentucky, Lexington.

Sloan, R. S. (1999). Guarded alliance relationships between hemodialysis patients and their healthcare providers. *American Nephrology Nurses' Association Journal, 26*(5), 503–505.

Sloan, R. S., Junod, S., Potter, M., & Ventrello, L. (1999, July 16). *Caring practices across nursing specialty areas: Recognizing invisibility.* Paper presented at the 3rd Biennial International Nursing Conference, The New Nursing: Converging Conversations of Education, Research, and Practice, Madison, WI.

Sloan, R. S., Kastan, B., Rice, S. I., Sallee, C. W., Yuenger, N . J., Smith, B., Ward, R. A., Brier, M. E., & Golper, T. A. (1998). Quality of life during and between hemodialysis treatments: The role of L-carnitine supplementation. *American Journal of Kidney Diseases, 32*(2), 265–272.

Sloan, R. S., & Rice, S. I. (2000). Legacies, liars and those alone: Lived experiences of end stage renal disease revealed through group work. *Journal of Nephrology Social Work 20*, 7–15.

Soskolne, V., & De-Nour, A. K. (1989). The psychosocial adjustment of patients and spouses to dialysis treatment. *Social Science and Medicine, 29*(4), 497–502.

Strauss, A. L. (1975). *Chronic illness and the quality of life.* St. Louis, MO: C. V. Mosby Company.

U.S. Renal Data Systems. (1997). *USRDS 1997 Annual Data Report.* Bethesda, MD: National Institutes of Health, National Institutes of Diabetes and Digestive and Kidney Diseases.

U.S. Renal Data Systems. (1998). *USRDS 1998 Annual Data Report.* Bethesda, MD: National Institutes of Health, National Institutes of Diabetes and Digestive and Kidney Diseases.

U.S. Renal Data Systems. (1999). *USRDS 1999 Annual Data Report.* Bethesda, MD: National Institutes of Health, National Institutes of Diabetes and Digestive and Kidney Diseases.

Wicks, M. N., Milstead, E. J., Hathaway, D. K., & Cetingok, M. (1997). Subjective burden of quality of life in family caregivers of patients with end stage renal disease. *American Nephrology Nurses' Association Journal, 24*(5), 527–538.

Yerby, J., Buerkel-Rothfuss, N., & Bochner, A. P. (1995). *Understanding family communication* (2nd ed.). Scottsdale, AZ: Gorsuch Scarisbrick Publishers.

4

The Violence of the Everyday in Healthcare

Elizabeth Smythe

Introduction

Power, oppression, and violence in healthcare: I put the words aside. They are too aggressive, too distasteful. They are not part of my world. My research did not go there. Months later the words are put to me again. This time I dwell on them a little longer as if to convince myself of the empowerment, emancipation, and nurturing that is part of the healthcare I know. And then the story of the shower comes to my mind. I am suddenly aware that I do have a contribution to make to this discussion. My doctoral study asked the question, "What is the meaning of being safe in childbirth?" I interviewed midwives, doctors, and women. Of all the stories, many of which were very moving, this was the one that had the greatest impact on me at the time, and this is the one which lives with me in my everyday world.

The woman had just told me about her long and difficult labor experience. Although her plan for a natural birth had not happened, although the forceps delivery had left her with a feeling that the birth "happened to her body" rather than that she had "given birth," she could accept that experience as being okay for that was how it needed to be. When she asked me if she should tell me what happened next, it was then that the tears came:

The morning after the birth, I couldn't move. I had had an epidural. I knew there was some sort of pad under me, but apart from that I really didn't know what they had done down there or what was happening or if I was bleeding everywhere or if I'd had an accident or what had happened, and I was actually quite scared of that. A nurse came in; I am sure she wasn't a midwife. They changed shifts. I said, "I need to go the toilet." She said I could go and have a shower and did I need a wheelchair? I said, "I don't know." So I sort of stood up and discovered that my legs worked vaguely and I said, "Oh I will walk down there to go to the loo." I actually got down there, and I was really upset because I didn't know what I could do and what I couldn't do. I knew I had stitches, and I didn't know if it would hurt when I went to the toilet. There are all those sorts of things that you don't know. And so in the end I called her on the buzzer and I said, "What can I do and what can't I do and I didn't pack soap and shampoo in my sponge bag, I don't know why." And she said, "Oh, well, I will get you some hospital soap." So she gave me some soap. It was a bit of a drama. I had forgotten my shampoo and so I said, "Look I'll just use soap." And I said, "What do I use to wash myself?" And she said, "Oh just wash yourself with water and you can use soap and all the rest of it." I actually needed a bit more "being with" than I got. She literally disappeared while I sort of struggled through a shower, and by the time I finished that, I collapsed. I got halfway back and they put me in a wheelchair and took me back to bed.

Looking back on that shower, I was petrified. I didn't actually feel particularly well, probably because I was hungry and that was probably the reason I didn't feel well, rather than I was losing heaps of blood or anything. And the other thing was I was terrified of leaving blood on their towel, and I was trying to avoid it. When I actually called, when I buzzed her to come back I burst into tears. I think then she realized how desperate I was and sort of did an about-face and stopped treating me a bit like a number and started talking to me. That was a really vulnerable time.

This woman, who the day before had bravely endured so much, was reduced to tears through the experience of having a shower. The impact of this story for me was that I could so easily have been that nurse. In the midst of a busy day I could have simply seen it as a task to be done. I could have expected that she would know what to do. I could have gotten frustrated that she didn't have any soap or shampoo because women are told they need to bring their own. I would never have imagined that she would be worried about getting blood on the towel. It just gets thrown into the dirty laundry at the end of the shower. I might have even thought (if I had stopped to think) that this woman would probably appreciate a bit of privacy after the very public experience of a forceps birth.

If this woman had not burst into tears, the nurse would never had known how she was feeling. The violence she was unknowingly committing would have remained hidden, covered over. Even with the tears, I wonder if this nurse appreciated the harm she had caused. Did she explain it to herself as the emotions of the postpartum experience? For me, it raises the question "what is the violence of everyday practice that goes by unnoticed, hidden, and caught up in the taken-for-grantedness of what we do?" For the woman who told me her story, the hurt of the unnamed violence brings her to tears a year later. How much unnamed violence goes on in the everyday world of practice? How does it linger with the people who are left feeling that some sort of violence has been done to them? My sense is that they themselves do not name it violence. They are more likely to simply carry the memories of the experience. The "violence," therefore, becomes covered over, hidden. There is no call to redress it. This study seeks to bring voice to that call.

Yet, what of the nurse who took this woman to the shower? Was she "being violent," or was she completing one of many tasks demanded of her? Was she frustrated that in a cost-cutting environment there was no hospital shampoo to offer this woman to enable her to better enjoy her post-birth shower? This study, therefore, also looks beyond the stories of violence to consider the possibility that health practitioners are themselves victims of violence, the violence of the entrapment of not having enough time or resources to enable caring.

The Phenomenon of the Violence of Everyday

The notion that will guide this study is "the phenomenon of the violence of everyday." Heidegger explains a phenomenon as "that which shows itself in itself" (1995, p. 5). I am looking for that which is perceived by the person having the experience as violence. I am looking for it "in itself," recognizing that it may show itself as a semblance, "as something which in itself it is not" (p. 51). For example, there may be a semblance of "being professional" hiding what is in itself uncaring, unthoughtful behavior. Or, there may be a semblance of violence that is in fact inflicting pain for "the good of," that is not in itself violence but care. Heidegger places emphasis on the need to "bring to the light of day, to put in the light" (p. 51). This means that the thing itself (everyday violence) is not yet in the light. It does, however, show itself in things that indicate. For example, in the story of the shower the woman's tears indicated something was not right. The tears themselves were not the phenomenon of "experiencing violence," they were a showing of what lay hidden, which may or may not have been an experience of violence. The woman herself gave some announcing of "the thing itself." She says she was "petrified . . . terrified . . . desperate . . . really vulnerable." In this bringing forth, the light is shed on her experience. I take her words, and from them I see a picture of everyday violence. It is not violence that is deliberate. It is rather violence that is so undeliberate that it is not even perceived as "being there" by the person providing "care." Yet, maybe, further hidden from sight is the entrapment of the practitioner who acts out care in a climate dictated by business ethos where the economic healthcare equation of efficiency, effectiveness, and evaluation by measurable outcomes undermines the heart of caring (Doncliff, 2000). It could be that the very nature of working in such a climate breeds violence that is experienced by both practitioner and client. Thus, the complexity of what lies hidden will be explored.

The Nature of the Quest

Heidegger (1995) explains that when we uncover and bring phenomena to the light we put our understanding into discourse, just as I have brought you the words "everyday violence." He calls the bringing together a synthesis, as letting the thing itself be seen in its "togetherness [*Beisammen*] with something—letting it be seen as something" (p. 56). He reminds us, however, that the "letting-something-be-seen" (p. 56) may be true or false. It may be that in this interpretive study I pass off the phenomenon of everyday violence "as something which it is *not*" (p. 57). Kaelin (1989) interprets these notions of Heidegger: "In true discourse . . . what gets talked about becomes revealed (*apophainsethai*) and becomes open to our simple, sensuous grasping as *aisthēsis* a seeing, hearing, perceiving. *Logos* [our discourse] as synthesis, and as possibly true or false, permits something to be seen as something" (p. 36).

Therein lies the tension before me. I have been called by a notion that there exists, hidden in the world of practice, a phenomenon of everyday violence. I perceive it to go unnoticed, unnamed, and thus unexamined. I seek to bring it to the light, to bring it forth, to show it as something to be seen as everyday violence. Yet, in the showing I may offer a semblance that is not the thing in itself. I may create a synthesis that is not a togetherness of everyday violence. I may name the thing in itself with language that is false. Maybe "violence" is too aggressive, too directive and has within it an inappropriate sense of deliberateness, yet, maybe we tend to ignore violence in its more subtle form.

My exploration within the *Oxford English Dictionary* (OED) (1970) reveals examples of the word violence being used in a similar manner to that proposed in this study. Perhaps closest is a quotation from Hammond (1649): "A kind of constraining and violencing of the spirit" (OED, p. 222). Note how in this example violence is portrayed in its "being" as violencing, a word no longer in common use. Another quote that spoke to me was from Caussin's Angel Peace 6 (1650): "The most Sacred things are violenced, and the most Profane are licenced" (OED, p. 222). This meaning rests with that which suffers violence, signifying the consequences of the act. A further quote by Yeowell (1847) shed light on what violence can be done to: "The first Christian missionaries in Ireland seem to have carefully avoided all unnecessary violence to the ancient habits of the aborigines" (OED, p. 221). To understand the habits of people is to understand them in their being. It seems that while violence is well known as a referent for physical force, it also has a close association with a more general sense of inflicting harm, as seen in a quote from Pusey (1860): "They did violence to the majesty of the law, . . . and then, through profaning it, did violence to man" (OED, p. 221). The meaning of the word is rich with possibilities.

The problematic nature of the quest of this study must lie open, or the study will in itself do violence in taking the reader to an unwarranted understanding. Let me be clear, the word *violence* is leading us on this exploration. The context in which I have chosen to explore it is within everyday practice. The examples I seek are those that have never before been named as violent, and those that harm the spirit or the being of a person. It is the violence that has few visible hallmarks by which it may be observed. It tends to lie hidden, unknown, yet perhaps known by us all.

The Methodology

The methodology I bring is informed by dialogues with the work of Martin Heidegger (1889–1976). Heidegger drew philosophy away from the metaphysical drive to "provide a universal, causal and logical account of Being" (Grondin, 1995, p. 10). For example, a more metaphysical perspective would consider violence as a theoretical concept and seek to describe its characteristics for all people at all times in all ways. Heidegger led philosophy into the quest to understand the being of notions like violence, in the experience of self, who is always there in the world, with others, in time. Heidegger further states that meaning will be found "within the horizon of average everydayness" (1995, p. 94) for that is where the self experiences being there. From this philosophical perspective comes also the awareness that interpretation is "grounded in something we have in advance" (Heidegger, 1995, p. 191). My interpretation, therefore, is grounded in my experiences as a nurse, a midwife, a teacher, a hermeneutic researcher, a citizen of New Zealand, and so the list could go on. I can only understand through my own understanding, which will always be different from the reader's. I seek to offer an uncovering of the nature of the violence of the everyday, not a generalizable truth.

Lawler (1998) suggests that in interpretive phenomenology there is a tendency for philosophy to overpower methodology. I argue that to draw from the writings of Heidegger is a "being with" experience. There is much more than guidance on how to approach the quest to understand. Because his writing focuses on the meaning of being in so many of its possibilities, there is always something in his writing to bring to an interpretation. I do not own to understanding Heidegger as he himself would want to be understood, but even in my glimmers of understanding, I come to see more about the nature of everyday violence than I would without his words to prompt my understandings. His writings, therefore, are always already there, alongside and within my interpretations. Sometimes I make this explicit with a specific reference, while at other times his notions simply become interwoven with my own thinking. I have been challenged that such an approach to research puts more emphasis on justifying Heidegger than on uncovering the meaning within the data. I see it as being more in the nature of the hermeneutic circle (Gadamer, 1982). As I take my interpretations from the data to my reading of Heidegger's work, I come to understand them in a new way, and as I understand how a story from the data reveals the nature of being, then I come to a deeper understanding of the notions described by Heidegger. Neither takes precedence. The data, the writings of Heidegger, my own groundings of understanding, my experience, and the input from colleagues all come together in the hermeneutic circle that brings forth interpretation.

The Method

The assumption that leads the data-gathering for this study is that if there is an undercurrent of violence existing in the everyday world of healthcare, then that undercurrent may announce itself, or make appearances, or show semblances in the research studies that already sit on the shelf. Without even looking, I knew it was there in my own doctoral study, from my interviews with practitioners and women about the meaning of being safe in childbirth (Smythe, 1998). I already had a close acquaintance with the research studies that sat on my own shelf. I selected five other studies to become the data for this study, all of a phenomenological–hermeneutic approach (Gasquoine, 1996; Madjar, 1998; Paddy, 2000; Spence, 1999; Thompson, 1999). The combination of studies spans the professions of nursing, midwifery, occupational therapy, and medical radiation technology (MRT). Three studies involve consumers and one students. One study is set in a community context, while the others mainly reflect a hospital setting. All are New Zealand studies. Savage (2000) offers the reminder that a research text does not offer a single unified meaning but is open to further interpretation. The research texts of these six studies are reinterpreted by means of a new question.

All of these studies are already in the public domain. I am mindful that none of the participants specifically gave consent to have their stories examined for examples of everyday violence. Therefore, I ask, is this study ethical? Van Manen (1990) calls phenomenology respectful. It is my intention to maintain respectfulness. I have the permission and enthusiastic support of the researchers to include data from their studies and have engaged their feedback through the writing process. The notion of the everydayness of violence resonated with them. Most of them identified the stories I will use. I take the stance that the participants themselves told their stories so that others may understand, and from that understanding, practice may improve. I believe this further examination of participants' stories gives them another opportunity to have their voices heard. I only know the identity of my own participants and remain committed to keeping identifying details secret. The anonymity of the participants from all the other studies has already been guarded against potential disclosure. There is no data to store safely, for all data are already in the public arena. The questions remains, is this study ethical? That question should not be ticked off as "approved" but remain open throughout.

Scanning the Literature

All of these studies were conducted in New Zealand. I searched the literature to find suggestions that the phenomenon of everyday violence may be endemic to healthcare throughout the world. In Kahn's (1999) ethnographic study of American nursing homes for older Jewish people I find glimpses of the hiddenness of such violence. The participants talk of "making the best of it." Kahn perceives them as downplaying the negative. Is it that they do not feel safe to expose the everyday violence of institutional care? A Swedish study by Soderberg, Lundman, and Norberg (1999) reveals the experience of women who suffer from fibromyalgia. They tell of what it is like to have an illness that is invisible, of how they are not believed, not taken seriously, not respected as human beings. One participant described perceiving herself to be thought of by practitioners as an ant. Are these appearances of everyday violence? Presumably the health professionals they came into contact with saw themselves as caring, nonviolent people. Yet, these women were left with feelings of hurt. Had they experienced the phenomenon of everyday violence?

A study into the experience of living with diabetes and hypertension in the southern United States (Weiss & Hutchinson, 2000) reveals the tension between deliberate violence and unintended violence. These people talked of the fear they experienced when they were warned by practitioners about what would happen to them if they did not follow treatment. Were the warnings deliberately intended to shock the client into a change of lifestyle, or did the practitioners have no idea of the fear they induced by describing the progress of the disease? Is it acceptable to invoke violence if it is ultimately in the best interests of the client? It seems likely, however, that there is violence in our communications with clients of which practitioners are unaware. An English study (Smith & Daughtrey, 2000) confirms the violence within client–practitioner communication. They share the story of a person who, an hour after discharge, is telephoned with the result of a test and assured that they can ring back anytime. "Yet in the space of 2 hours [when I phoned for advice] it seemed it was not their problem anymore" (p. 818).

An appearance of violence is also revealed in a study that describes the practitioner perspective. Castellani and Wear (2000) interviewed physicians about their experience of practice professionalism in the corporate age. Words that appear in the discussion are: "attacks," "clash," "threat," "intimidation," "distraught," "under siege," "overturned," "yanked." The perception of violence is close below the surface. These practitioners are no longer free to practice as they think best. They must practice within constraints imposed upon them, and I suggest they experience the violence that is within that restraint.

Returning to the New Zealand literature, I find a research study by Opie (1998), exploring the clients' experience of empowerment (or, more to the point, disempowerment) by multidisciplinary health teams. She tells the story of Mrs. Edgar. In a 20-minute meeting about plans for her discharge, Mrs. Edgar speaks up twice. Both times she is ignored or overruled. The professionals decide for her. She is marginalized and silenced. How might Mrs. Edgar still be feeling about that experience? What is it like to have health professionals take over the decisions about where you will live? Is it possible to be truly concerned for the welfare of another if one ignores the dissent of that person? From Opie's study I suggest that everyday violence happens when health professionals "seem" to operate "in the best interests of the client" when in fact the true interests are more likely to be those of the institution or the family.

Clarifying the Phenomenon

This scanning of the literature has confirmed that both clients and practitioners experience episodes that could be those of everyday violence. The phenomenon I seek is not about the violence that brings tangible harm. If I hit someone, the act itself can be witnessed, or the bruise can provide evidence of harm. Such violence is more likely to be already "in the light" or able to be brought "to the light" by those who are harmed. It is also not the violence of abuse, where the perpetrator is aware of his or her actions and in that awareness takes care to keep both the actions and the consequences hidden. The violence this study seeks to illuminate is the violence that is only known by the person receiving it. At the time of its happening it is likely to be seen by witnesses as part of everyday practice. They may perceive it to be average or poor practice, but they are unlikely to step in and put a stop to it. It would be simply taken for granted as being "how things are."

Understanding "Self"

To understand such violence we must look to the "self." It is only the self who can experience it, understand it, and live with it. How then does Heidegger explain the self? My reading of *Being and Time* (Heidegger, 1995) makes the following interpretation. The self cannot be separated or divorced from the context in which he or she is situated. As self one is already there, already in sickness or health, already happy or sad or something in between. People are who they are because of the situation in which they find themselves. Heidegger says that being is "co-determined" (p. 153). If one is angry, one is not simply angry; rather, one is angry because someone or something, in presence or absence, in what happens or does not happen, has provoked anger. The world, the *Dasein*, or being-there-in the-world cannot be avoided. It is as it is. It is a world always shared by others. I can only understand self in relation to how others affect my notions of self. If they affirm me, treat with respect, take heed of my opinion, enable me to be who I want to be, then I am likely to feel good about myself. If, on the other hand, they scorn me, laugh at me, ignore me, and override my wishes, then I experience myself as disgruntled, frustrated, and cross. Others do not even have to be present to have this affect on me. On one occasion being left alone may be interpreted by me as the other having confidence in my ability. On another occasion, aloneness may be frightening, and I may be annoyed at the person who is not there to help me.

The Nature of Concern

Heidegger (1995) goes on to explain that we need to understand being there with others in terms of care or concern. He lists the attributes of concern as: having to do with something, producing something, attending to something and looking after it, making use of something, giving something up and letting go, undertaking, accomplishing, evincing, interrogating, considering, discussing, determining. One could make the assumption that all these activities are done for the good of the client, or the colleague, or the person one is in relationship with. But recall the story of Mrs. Edgar (from Opie's study, 1998). She was at the mercy of such concern that sought to "do to." She did not experience the health team's behaviors toward her as concern.

From the shower story at the beginning of this paper is the cry for concern: "I needed a bit more 'being with' than I got" (Smythe, 1998, p. 210). Heidegger goes on to explain two extreme possibilities of concern's positive mode. One he calls "leaping in," where care is taken away from the other, where, like Mrs. Edgar, the other is taken over. Leaping in may have kept Mrs. Edgar physically safe, but it did not necessarily make her feel safe. Heidegger calls the other mode of concern "leaping ahead," where one goes ahead of the other, not to take their care away but to give it back to them. The woman in the shower story may have enjoyed the aloneness if the nurse had first explained, answered her questions, and given her confidence. Once in her state of vulnerability, however, she needed someone to leap in and tell her what to do. She needed someone to be right there, attending to her, helping her, telling her, encouraging her. The complexity of concern is revealed in the stories where the leaping in should have been leaping ahead and vice versa. It may be that it is not the task itself that determines the mode of care but the mood of the person at the time. If a person is feeling vulnerable there is likely to be a hope for care and understanding. However, if a person is feeling strong and independent, then approaches of nurturance may be interpreted as unnecessary interference. Perhaps, when we get it wrong, the person experiences a sense of violence. That is, when we leap in inappropriately the person feels taken over and dominated. When we leap ahead when the person is feeling vulnerable and in immediate need, they feel stranded. The challenge is to first attune to the person's mood, for it may reveal the need.

Further to the possibility of not matching the nature of our concern with the person's mood, Heidegger tells us that the nature of people is that they are not always concerned. For the most part, he suggests we are "there" in indifferent or deficient modes where we may not care much, or not care at all, or not even recognize that there is a need to care. He describes such modes as characterizing "everyday, average Being-with-one-another" (1995, p. 158).

This, then, is where we are most likely to find the violence of everyday. It will be in situations when the "someone," for whatever reason, is no longer in the attuned mode of caring and instead offers indifferent or negligent care. Or, it may be in situations where the mode of leaping has been misjudged.

Turning to the Data

If self is a codetermined understanding, how does self meet the other? What greets them? What reaches out and impacts them? These are the questions I bring to the data.

Not Wanted

The first story is from a mother whose son was hospitalized for asthma. The medical ward was full, so they were admitted to a surgical ward.

We turned up and weren't wanted. . . . I think we were a bit . . . sort of slightly alien there, aliens there because we didn't really belong to that ward and they were doing it as a special favour to the other ward. (Gasquoine, 1996, p. 72)

This woman, anxious for her son, wanting the best care for her son, arrived to the place of care to be greeted by a sense of "not being wanted." She felt alien, an outsider, somebody who did not belong. She talks of "we," indicating that her child in the midst of an episode of asthma was made to feel the same. I cannot imagine any of the staff who greeted them thinking to themselves, "Let's make it clear to these people that they are not wanted here." Rather, I imagine staff confused and thrown out of their normal routines, not being able to work with their ready-to-hand confidence (Heidegger, 1995). Instead of an embodied sense of caring, they would have to stop and think. Maybe they felt nervous about the medications, maybe they felt apprehensive about the nature of asthma itself. Maybe their ward was busy, and they felt hard done by having to also take on the work of another ward. Whatever the feelings that underpinned their welcome of this mother and son, I suggest that the staff would have had no idea that in this time of these people needing care, they made them feel not wanted. Is this an example of the violence of everydayness? It fits with the notion of violence only known by those that received it. It is violence that would pass unnoticed by the providers of care. Yet, let us call this assumption to question. How does it feel to be thrown out of one's normal mode of practice? Was there violence to the staff of this ward who were put in a situation of not being able to "give of their best"? The woman who told this story used the word "alien." One definition of alien is "out of harmony" (Sykes, 1985). When the harmony is lost there is discord. I suggest all the players in the story were experiencing discord. The jarring, clashing harshness of discord could be likened to a climate of violence.

Not Being Understood

From my study on being safe in childbirth comes a woman's story of the practitioners she met in the midst of her experience of miscarriage:

I had a miscarriage with my first pregnancy. It wasn't a planned baby, and I was surprised at how upset I was when it happened. It was very traumatic. I had a scan and they said, "Look there is nothing there. You might believe, or your body thinks you are three months pregnant, but there is nothing." In the end we phoned the guy on call at my local GP [General Practitioner Doctor] who was such a dick. Here I was reeling around in agony, I wanted to take all my clothes off. I don't know if that's an autonomic response. I just wanted to get everything off me. I felt I just wanted to pace and walk around. I was hot and thought I was going to vomit. And he kept sort of trying to counsel me about having a miscarriage, "How do you feel about this?" It was just so inappropriate. I mean, I didn't want to talk about that right then. I just wanted to get rid of that pain. He gave me a jab in my leg, then I went really way out. I went to hospital for a D&C [Dilatation & Curettage]. There was a Doctor there who kept quizzing me. He said something, and I responded in such a way that he seemed to be horrified. I think I said, "I just want to get this out of me, I just want to get rid of it." He looked appalled that I would say such a thing. After the D&C, I woke up and it was gone, it was absolutely gone, the pain was gone. I felt great. I said, "Well, I want to go home." I had to wait for another couple of hours because I'd had an anaesthetic, and then I said, "I want to go home, I feel fine." The nurse understood, she was very nice. But it was a bad experience, it was a really bad experience. (Smythe, 1998, p. 123)

In the midst of agonizing pain and huge emotional upset, this woman was greeted by two different doctors, each of whom gave a semblance of caring. The first recognized the emotional trauma of the experience and took it upon himself to leap ahead with the woman to help her deal with the consequences of the loss. Right then, all the woman could think about was trying to cope with the pain. All she needed and wanted was someone to leap in and give her pain relief. He was an extra stress she needed to cope with. The second doctor at the hospital seemed also to be in leap-ahead mode with the questions he thought needed to be asked. The woman just wanted to get the experience over with. She didn't want any quizzing. When she voiced her raw feelings of wanting to "get this out of me," "get rid of it," she recalls him looking appalled. Now, as well as her own distress, she was given the impression that she was a terrible woman for wanting to get rid of her baby. She remembers this look at the interview some 4 years later. I imagine that both these doctors felt they were doing their job well. Both made efforts to assist this woman in her time of need. Both, however, got it wrong and left her with lasting memories that perhaps she should have handled this miscarriage in a manner more caring of her loss.

Did they get it wrong because they were insensitive to her mood, or was it that their sensitivities did not have the luxury of time to dwell and to wait? Was this their one encounter with this woman, which therefore pressured them into expressing all their concerns while they were there? Does the fragmented, allocated, prescriptive nature of institutional practice lead to behaviors that are efficient rather than attuned? Is, perhaps, efficiency a double-sided coin, the face-down side being violence?

Someone got it right. When she said she wanted to go home, the nurse did not try to dissuade her or check out if it was a good idea. She simply understood. But then, could it be that in the era of cost-cutting, staff are encouraged to get patients out of hospital as soon as they are able. Were the woman's needs and the hospital's need simply in accord? Can caring sometimes be a semblance for expediency?

Not Liking

The woman in the story above reported that the nurse was nice. In Paddy's (2000) study there is a description from a client about a community occupational therapist who was also measured against the word "nice":

I've had dealings with another occupational therapist from another service. I have a great aversion to this person who I didn't like at all. She was very intrusive and quite rude. She asked all these questions as though she didn't believe me, and it felt like she was trying to catch me out [in a lie] all the time. I think personality had a lot to do with it and she needed a personality transplant. There was nothing nice about her. She was brusque, she was abrupt, and she was sharp. There was no relaxing with her. (p. 74)

This therapist was not nice, there was nothing nice about her. She was intrusive, rude, brusque, and sharp. The woman was made to feel as though she were not believed, as though she were being tricked into telling the truth. Such a meeting was a stressful experience. The woman explains such behavior as belonging to the woman's personality and suggests a "personality transplant." Does the therapist carry with her pre-understandings that clients are not to be believed, or is this tension unique to this relationship? From this client's perspective it seems she sees it as her duty to get to the bottom of the matter by whatever means it takes. She is not caring for the person, perhaps rather caring about the tasks that need to be done. While she is "there with" she is not engaged in the "withness."

Whose responsibility is such violence of practice? Assuming that the therapist herself is indifferent to the stress she engenders in this client, then who should care enough to stop this assault? Is it that in community practice where the therapist relates to clients in their own homes, there are no colleagues to witness or temper such behavior? The hiddenness could be one of not-being-seen. Yet, as I write this, I recall colleagues of a similar personality whose practice I have seen and ignored. Could it be that in professional practice there is also a hiding away of what we see but wish we had not seen for it seems too hard to do anything about? Does a climate in which violence reveals itself also give rise to a fear in the colleagues who must continue to work with such people?

Being Judged

Returning to my own study, there is a story of a client feeling judged by a midwife:

After our homebirth my baby needed to be admitted to SCBU [Special Care Baby Unit] because of some degree of respiratory distress, and I was admitted to the postnatal ward. I don't know how much of it was my anticipation of being treated like that and how much of it was actually being treated like that, but you know this sort of business of "silly woman, fancy having homebirth, of course this was going to happen," to the point where the following day one of the midwives on the postnatal ward, whose care I had been allocated to, saying, "Oh yes, now you are the failed homebirth aren't you?" Absolutely extraordinary, and she didn't have any idea why I was in there. I remember her saying, "Well why are you here?" (Smythe, 1998, p. 185)

This professional woman had responsibly planned and experienced a very successful homebirth. Following birth, her baby was required to be admitted for special care. The place of birth made no difference to the care this baby now required. In New Zealand 5% of babies are born at home (The National Health Committee, 1999). Homebirth is an accepted choice of childbirth, yet it is still shrouded in myths of unsafety. This woman felt some apprehension about coming into hospital following a homebirth. Her fears were justified. As a new mother, with her baby experiencing respiratory distress, she was told she was "the failed homebirth." She was labeled, with all the connotations that go with the label (irresponsible, foolish, and a failure). This woman felt totally misjudged. From where did the off-the-tongue label of failed homebirth spring? It suggests that in everyday practice there are discourses that place unfair and misleading judgments on people. Such judgments hurt. It placed this woman, who was already in a situation of concern for her baby, in the added situation of having to prove that she was a responsible mother who was not a failure. She did not need that call upon her energies. She did not need the label etched upon her memory.

There is, however, the thought that this midwife did not recognize the power of the words she used, but was she unthinkingly repeating the discourse of the institution? Perhaps violence is endemic in the language of everyday practice.

Being Forgotten

Another mother describes a vulnerable memory from when her baby was hospitalized:

I was going to bath Robert about the second or third day, and he still had the oxygen tubes up his nose and you know all this sort of stuff and I told my nurse that I was going to do this and she said I'll be back to help but of course she didn't come back and I sort of left it and left it and thought oh look I have got to do it, you know, and I didn't feel I could ring and ask her . . . or go out and ask and say look I am going to bath the baby do you want to give me a hand, because I did feel I needed a hand.

(What was it you needed help with?) It was *support!* . . . Support, just so as I knew I wasn't going to rip something out which . . . or just an extra pair of hands to hold the towel or whatever . . . I mean he was a new baby.

Also he was floppy. And then I didn't want to not bath him either. I mean I could have just said oh well I won't bath him it is no big hassle, but I didn't because I felt maybe that . . . I mean it was something that I wanted to do with him I think. You know—I wanted to be normal (Gasquoine, 1996, p. 78).

This mother was going to bathe her baby. You can feel her anticipation coming through this story; after some anxious days she was now going to do something for her baby that was a "normal" part of her role as "mother." It was to be about much more than cleaning his skin. Yet, it was going to be a much more complicated exercise than a normal bath because of his condition and all the tubes. The nurse said she would come back and help. Note the way the woman says "but of course she didn't." It is almost as though it was too much to expect the nurse to do that, too much to hope that the busy nurse would be able to simply be there and give support. The woman is left waiting and hoping, wrestling with her dilemma. What was to be an important reclaiming of her mothering role has instead become a huge stress as she is confronted with her own sense of inadequacy. The idea of ringing the bell, or asking for help, reinforces the tension within her that she perhaps shouldn't need help or that bathing wasn't important.

And what of the nurse? She might have simply forgotten, she might have been called to more important tasks. It is most unlikely that she left that room thinking, "I will keep that woman waiting and stewing all day, I will not help her." It may be that she spent her day trying to get back and carried with her the sense of having let the woman down. This is one of those situations common to the everydayness of practice when intentions are not fulfilled. King (1964, p. 81) interprets Heidegger in saying in the world people are "pressed upon and hemmed in." It is likely that this nurse was pressed upon and hemmed in by other demands on her time and on her mind. Meanwhile, this mother suffered. The violence was perpetrated by the caring phrase, "I'll be back to help." The nurse, also, may have been haunted by those words, knowing she had not met her promise. Is it timely to voice concern that the health-care environment has taken the "hope of help" from both the client and the nurse?

Being Interrogated

It seems that so many of the stories in this study are about what could easily be described as "good practice." Consider this next story.

The woman is describing her observations from being in a four-bedded room in an antenatal ward. This woman had premature rupture of the membranes at 21 weeks with a twin pregnancy. There was never anything to see when she visited her own doctor, so he did nothing. After revisiting him several times he finally referred her to hospital:

There was one thing I found all the way through is that all the doctors, this is no one's particular fault, like everyone was the same, and I noticed that they did it to other women that were in the ward as well, is that they all go now, "What was it like? What colour was it? What was this like? What was that like?" They try to get you in your ignorant way to describe what you have seen, and they won't actually look at it themselves. As soon as one nurse actually said, "Well, can I just have a look at your pad," and she goes, "Oh, that is liquor" [amniotic fluid indicating ruptured membranes]. And you just think 'ohh'. They did it to another girl who was in the other bed and she had sort of bleeding. They were trying to decide whether she had ruptured her membranes, and they kept on asking her, "Well what does it look like?" because it was only happening every so often. She would go, "Well it is sort of like . . . ," and they would say, "Well how much is it?," and it is really hard to decide how much and what colour and all this sort of thing. Once she went up to a nurse and showed her, and the nurse looked at her as if she was some really weird person. I thought it would be much easier if they could just like look and say, "Oh that is what it is," or "this is old blood or new blood or this size or this amount," because they should know. (Smythe, 1998, p. 193)

This woman had experienced several weeks of not being believed. She had tried her best to describe the fluid that was draining from her, but without seeing it for themselves, no one would take her descriptions as "being true" or specific enough for the nurse to make the qualitative distinctions (Benner, Tanner, & Chesla, 1996) that were sought. Finally a nurse asks to look at the pad and, with the voice of authority, is able to declare that it is "liquor." Hear the frustration of the woman as she made the "ohh" response. How must that feel? The woman goes on to describe her observations of other women's experiences. How can you describe something when you have never before seen the "thing in itself" and therefore do not have the words to put to the thing? How do you know the difference between old and new blood if no one has ever explained how to tell the difference? How do you explain the amount of discharge when it is all soaked into a pad? What does it feel like to be asked questions about the thing you are most worried about when you do not have the language that seems to tell? I share this woman's puzzlement of why language was expected to achieve what the eyes of the practitioner could have much more effectively ascertained. Weren't the nurses' questions in this case directed toward finding that understanding—giving the patient words to describe what she saw?

Could it be, however, that these practitioners were being sensitive to the intimate nature of vaginal discharge and did not wish to do violence by intruding? Does the fear of "doing violence" constrain practitioners from looking for themselves? Yet, perhaps their questions were even more intrusive. They brought to the light "the issue" but left it unresolved and confused. Imagine the feelings of these "questioned" women as the doctors left the room. They knew they hadn't been able to tell them what they needed them to know. They were in hospital to receive care, but the care, even in its caring, had been wanting. When one woman tried to remedy this by showing the nurse her pad, she was looked at as though she was "some really weird person."

Note also that the woman telling this story was able to see the violence dealt to the other woman. In the with-world she was with-the-other as the questions were fired and the look was given. She saw the violence because she too felt its impact.

Why is there so much violence when the practitioners are trying to care and the women want to be cared for? Yet, this same woman told of one of the doctors coming to see her after the Caesarian section birth of her twins at 27 weeks gestation. One twin had died soon after birth because there had been no fluid around her even though the ultrasound scans had shown that "there were two sacs, that both had the same amount of fluid and they were both quite normal" (Smythe, 1998, p. 208). The woman describes the visit from the doctor:

The doctor came afterwards. He was really helpful all the way through. He had tears in his eyes. It made me cry just seeing the tears in his eyes. He said, "I'm sorry we couldn't have warned you what was going to happen." I said, "Well don't worry because I wouldn't have wanted to have known; this is the best way that it could have happened." (p. 208)

This woman had a deep sense of the caring of the doctor. He knew that they had unwittingly misled her into believing that the ruptured membranes had not caused problems. He was distressed that they had not been able to warn her. She knew however that the warning would have made it worse. This could have been told as a story of anger, yet it is clearly a story of care. Perhaps it was because the mother and the doctor shed tears together at the violence of losing a precious baby. Perhaps, also, the doctor saw afresh the limits of technology, at a time when all he could offer this woman was the humanity of sharing her sorrow. It is a story that brings hope that caring can prevail. One wonders, however, if it takes the tragedies of practice to displace efficiency with "being with."

Being Called To

The next story reveals the paradox of a client describing a nurse as doing violence by being caring:

After about half an hour or three quarters of an hour of being paced through [a dressing change], I felt I was becoming terribly tired, and I found it almost hard to concentrate on what she [nurse] was saying. . . . I really felt that I just wanted to be left with my head down and being able to close my eyes with nothing being said at all. . . . My tolerance level became a little low, and it was just like "Forget it! I just want the whole thing to be finished" at that stage . . . [having] to make answers, which took effort . . . a mental effort . . . tiring, very tiring. (Madjar, 1998, p. 111)

This nurse seems to have been concerned and caring. It is unlikely she had any notion of the effort she was demanding of this patient. All this patient wanted was to close her eyes and be in silence. Her wanting was a not wanting, not wanting the nurse to make an effort, not wanting to have to respond, not wanting to engage with the world. She therefore experiences the thoughtful conversation as violence. It invades her silence. It calls on her to make an effort. It drains her of her flagging energy. It is in this story that we find the everydayness of violence in the midst of the caring of care. It is the paradox of practice, where care becomes harm, even in the recognition that it is care.

Care can only be known as "care" from the experience of the person being cared for. Care as violence is a notion that needs to be considered in the act of giving care. It calls to question that one can ever assume to be caring, unless the meaning of what is "caring" is given over to the person being cared for. That means letting go of the assumptions of good intentions and being mindful that only the client knows the goodness of the experience of care.

Being Told

In Gasquoine's (1996) study one mother describes her experience of being given advice:

It was such a really terrifically hard choice to take their advice and wean him or whether I was doing the best thing by breast feeding, because it is what everybody says, breast feed, breast feed, you know until you drop just about. And I really thought I was doing the best thing because he loved it and that is all he would drink and you know he wouldn't take a bottle and it was really hard. (p. 83)

I imagine that the practitioners of this story must have had a good reason for advising this woman to give up breastfeeding. However, they left her in torment. Just as Heidegger (1995) talks of the dictatorship of the nameless, faceless "they" who dictate what we should and should not do, so this woman tells us of the "everybody" who would demand she keep breastfeeding. She wants the best for her baby, and she wants to do her best. She is left stretched between the two camps of authority. The very people whom she would expect to advise her to continue to breastfeed are telling her to stop.

Heidegger would further tell us that our primordial knowing comes from experience. This woman is experiencing a baby who loves breastfeeding and is breastfeeding well and seems to be sharing her own resistance to bottle feeding. There is clearly no intentional violence in this story, yet there is a picture of violence in the woman's account. How is it that, when practitioners seek to give sound advice, they put people into such a situation? Was their call to bottle feed the best decision? Best for whom? Did they understand what depriving the mother and baby of the breastfeeding experience would mean to them? Did they help the woman to come to her own understanding of the need to the change? Did they stop to ask any questions at all? Or had they agonized over the advice to stop breastfeeding but in the culture of professionalism, hid the tension of their decision? Is it questioning what is assumed to be right—by both the patient and nurse?

Being Asked to Give Too Much

The data reveal that it is not only the clients who experience violence but also the practitioners. A midwife in my study, who has her own caseload, was very open about the impact of clients on her life:

I've had quite a bad scene on lately of having clients that I've really found difficult. I get to the stage where I can't bear to go and see them sometimes, and I actually have to force myself to go and see them. And that's awful. It shouldn't be like that, and it's probably unsafe for the woman. I don't know how to best work out an escape clause. Like how do you say to someone at 32 weeks, "Look, I don't want to look after you any more". Doctors don't do that. It's not the same, is it. They see them in a consulting room for 2 minutes, for blood pressure, urine, and the physical type things. Women don't do those same things at doctors anyway. They don't unload it all. One or two of them that have been particularly difficult, I realise that they really wanted me to be their friend, and when it became apparent that I wasn't going to be their best friend, then the only thing I could be was an enemy. That's what I find the most difficult. I get quite intense about it, and I can't just laugh it off. Like I sit there and seethe with anger about them sometimes. I think they're just eating up my life. They don't seem to have any awareness that I've got children and a family, and I want to do other things as well. That I'll give my all to them, but I don't want them ringing me up four times a day to tell me inconsequential things. And then accuse me of being distant when I don't respond 100% enthusiastically. (Smythe, 1998, p. 203)

This midwife tells of the accumulation of feelings that have built up in her about clients. She has to force herself to go and see them. She doesn't want to continue in the relationship but doesn't know how to get out of it. She describes how the women "unload" everything on her. They are eating up her life and disturbing her home life unnecessarily with "inconsequential things." Sometimes she seethes with anger. She is aware of the difference of expectations and believes these women are looking for a best friend. When she fails to meet their expectations she senses they then see her as the enemy. It is heavy stuff. Metaphors of enemy demonstrate the level of violence she is feeling. What makes it worse is her sense of being trapped and at the same time knowing her feelings are not creating a safe relationship with her clients. She senses that, despite her efforts, the clients want more. This story reminds us that being a practitioner is about being human. Practitioners have feelings in response to client expectations and demands. When the client expects more than the practitioner is prepared or able to give, the practitioner may experience violence. This midwife notes how the women do not seem to have an awareness of how they intrude into her life. They rather interpret her unenthusiastic response as a "distance." How can a practitioner protect herself from such violence? Perhaps more importantly, how can the potential for violence in client–practitioner relationships be guarded against?

Violence, in a situation such as this, where the relationship is ongoing, has the likelihood of impacting on both parties. When there is distance, when there are perceptions of each being the enemy of the other, how can "concern for" override such feelings? The relationship is likely to be overtaken by a mere semblance of concern, while underneath the seething goes unabated.

This story, told by the practitioner rather than the client, again reminds us that always when client and practitioner come together there are expectations of relationship. Just as this midwife perceives women want her to be their best friend, so the previous stories have shown a call for wanting to belong, to be understood, to like and be liked, to be respected, to be remembered, to be believed, and to be cared for in the "right" way. They are big demands, and yet they are such simple expectations. They cost no money, but perhaps they all cost time and energy. How does a system that is structured for and rewards efficiency and effectiveness of interventions discourse on these "simple expectations?"

Being Robbed of Integrity

Another practitioner, this time a nurse, talks about her experience of having her integrity challenged:

It was really frustrating and I felt quite hurt. I was the person who got that brunt. I thought I'd tried really hard. It was a difficult relationship but I thought I had persevered well with it and it all came back to me . . . I had handed over, saying his luer [intra-venous cannula] needed to be re-sited. It was two shifts before I saw him again. . . . It wasn't managed satisfactorily for him and we do need to be accountable . . . I just felt my integrity had been challenged and that I didn't have an opportunity to defend myself. He was so angry he wasn't rational. I just had to swallow it and still be professional and cheerful towards him. He expected that. (Spence, 1999, p. 125)

This nurse did her best. In her absence, the management of the intra-venous cannula was not satisfactory. For whatever reason, this nurse got the blame and was not able to defend herself. The integrity that she valued had been robbed of her. She had to receive the anger with a professional, smiling face. Her sense of violence needed to be hidden, yet she carries it with her. It was not fair or just. Her sense of self had been re-interpreted by others in an inappropriate manner. A question is surfacing about the feelings practitioners carry with them in their everyday practice that have come from an experience of violence and linger with them. Heidegger reminds us that our past always goes ahead of us to meet us in the moment of now (1995). When a person feels misjudged, what impact might that have on their ongoing practice?

Being Scared

The next story is from a community occupational therapist. She describes the challenge of a particular relationship:

The main thing was that he did scare me when I first went in to see him. I felt like a little girl and I think that he looked at me as a little girl . . . [I] had a cold sweat whenever I went there and thought, oh my God am I going to say the right thing.

He could be very critical. What he wanted done he wanted done now and he wanted it done properly. It was almost like I proved myself to him. I proved that I actually could do the job and he respected that. (Paddy, 2000, p. 107)

This practitioner experienced the violence of being treated like she didn't know what she was doing, being criticized, and being expected to do things properly and promptly. Yet, this is another story of hope, for it shows a practitioner who cared enough to endure the cold sweats until finally she earned his respect for doing the job well.

The Cost of Caring

Another story from a community occupational therapist tells of what practice can feel like:

Often I come back in tears, once or twice anyway. I was just shocked really, especially the time I was really stressed out anyway. I realised that I needed to give myself a bit more time, more space when I needed it. . . . At times I had to use my senior therapist and other staff to unload to because of difficulties in the relating. (Paddy, 2000, p. 143)

The stories suggest that the difficulties in relating are experienced by both clients and practitioners. Time seems to be integral to both the experiencing of violence and the recovering from violence. When things go wrong, it seemed it was often because there was not enough time. More time might have led to better attunement, to taking the trouble to come to understand and to explain, to simply "being with." This person describes her need for the time to have space for herself. Just as her clients want her time, so she also recognizes that unless she sets aside time to give herself she becomes really stressed out. Time makes the difference. The metaphor of the business ethos reminds us that "time is money," yet I argue that these stories show that inadequate time also has its costs. The question is, how should cost be measured? Is there a measure more important than money? What is the measure of humanity's response to humanity?

Being Thrown In

Next is a story that reveals the relationship between the expert and the learner. It takes us back to the taken-for-granted situations that are part of everyday institutional life, this time told by a student:

I was involved in my first barium enema [examination to demonstrate the large intestine using barium, a dye] at the other placement and I said "look, I haven't done one of these before" and she [supervising Medical Radiation Technologist] said "this is all you have to do, this is the clamp, and talk to the patient" and then she went and stood behind the screen. I was horrified with this bag hanging midway in the air and with the patient there. I couldn't even say "it won't be long now, you're nearly finished," because I didn't know. I didn't know what was going to happen next, I mean the table was spinning everywhere, that's daunting enough. I had to fiddle around with all the buttons with him spinning everywhere and I kept on saying "the bands will hold you". I knew that much. Then the doctor said "can you drain it". No one had told me to stick it down at the side of the table. So when the bed started turning I'm there trying to hold onto the bag and the radiologist said to me "just leave it and let it hang" and I thought surely that can't be comfortable with this thing hanging so I picked it up and he said "no let it hang," so I let it go. I mean there was an expectation that you're a second year student, you should know, but it's quite different to where I'm from. Barium enemas hardly ever come through. (Thompson, 1999, p. 101)

Here we find the supervisor leaping ahead to tell the student what he needs to do, enabling him to do it for himself. Her teaching, however, is not enabling enough. In the midst of the experience the student realizes all that he does not know and has no way of knowing other than in experiencing it in itself. What is worse is that he witnesses the client's need for knowledge, and he has none to give him. The directions he receives from the doctor don't make sense, so he tries to work them out, but then gets the instructions repeated. I can sense both frustration and humiliation of the student in this situation. When people are thrown into experiences for the first time, they can never know the experience by the instructions alone for the experience will always be more than that. Those who are experienced may often overlook the vulnerability, the fear, and the violence that may accompany a first-time experience as a student. This supervisor no doubt thought she had prepared the student well and even afterwards may have felt comfortable about how she and the student had handled the situation. The doctor may have thought his instructions were helping, but for the student they were confusing. This experience is likely to remain with the student always as a "being thrown in the deep end" experience. It may have given him confidence that he can cope in such situations, but his horror and sense of helplessness seem to be the dominant memories. It calls for a mindfulness about violence that may be inflicted on a student, calling to question the manner in which experienced practitioners may effectively offer support. At the same time, it asks "what responsibilities do the education providers have to prepare the way?"

Being Within a System

It is important to recognize that both clients and practitioners are within a context of care which exerts its authority, dictates how things will be done, and at the same time exists in the chaos of the thrownness of being (Heidegger, 1995). While plans can be made, they may not be able to happen in an anticipated way. This story, told by an obstetrician, reveals how the system impacts on the woman's experience:

Nobody in our hospital, house surgeon or registrar level, can diagnose a miscarriage without having ultrasound scans. As a result I actually believe patients get worse treatment than they need, because they come into hospital at lunchtime one day, and they can't get an ultrasound appointment till 5 o'clock, and then somebody goes home, and then they have to have a full bladder so they drink a lot, and then it means they can't get to theatre [surgery] until 10 at night, and at 10 at night there are so many people waiting to go to theatre that they don't get done during the night, and they stay in hospital overnight, and eventually get to theatre after the morning lists the next day. They go home at 5 or 6 o'clock the second day, when in fact they should have been dealt with, and sent off, at 5 o'clock the first day. (Smythe, 1998, p. 170)

This story is told from the experience of how miscarriage used to be diagnosed before the era of ultrasound scanning for everyone. The obstetrician reveals the violence he feels on behalf of the women, who in a time of personal crisis are caught up in a system that keeps them waiting until they can be slotted in for a scan and then to theatre. Perhaps he experiences the violence because he is the one who must explain, or try to explain, why they need to wait. Further to his frustration is the trap that he suggests practitioners have made for themselves in coming to rely on scans, thereby losing both the clinical skills and the right to diagnose a miscarriage without a scan. The problem is no one person's fault. It is simply how the world of practice has evolved. The institutional climate of policies, rituals, and routines has entrapped both the practitioner and the client. The resulting violence is enacted in the momentum of "how things are done."

Waiting in Dread

Following an experience of violence, a woman tells of facing the ongoing meetings with her occupational therapist:

The minute she turned up all my barriers went up. I thought, here we go again. I am not one to make a fuss and I don't like to rock the boat . . . so I haven't complained. But I used to dread her coming. I really did. (Paddy, 2000, p. 148)

The violence stays with this woman as she dreads the next visit. She is not a person to complain. She uses the metaphor of "rocking the boat," implying that to complain might bring other unforeseen problems, so she simply waits in dread. When the therapist arrives, up go the barriers to protect her from the next onslaught of violence.

The Lingering of Violence

From Madjar's (1998) study comes this story of how one experience of violence to a patient experiencing pain lingered for a day:

It hurt. It definitely hurt. It's hard to describe how it hurt, but it did not have the same calming, soothing effect because I almost felt that she was in a hurry. She was coming from one patient to another, and to another, and I was one [of] perhaps five or six. . . . The feel was very rushed and not relaxed. I felt quite tense when she left here, and it took me actually quite a while to relax and get back into a relaxed state. Quite a while. I noticed that particularly today . . . it's had an effect on how badly I've tolerated pain. I haven't tolerated pain particularly well today . . . it just made me more uptight, made me more tense and therefore made it more difficult to cope. (p. 102)

The violence in this painful experience was one of being rushed. The patient knew from past experience that there could be a calming, soothing approach, which made the experience much easier to cope with. This time that was absent, and the rushing caused him to feel more and more tense. The tension stayed with him throughout the day and made it harder to cope with the pain. Violence sets up a mood of tension that lingers in the aftermath. It becomes the backdrop against which the rest of the challenges of the day must be dealt with.

Feeling Guilty

The next story reveals the subtleties of violence and its aftermath of guilt:

And up until then I had been using the staff quarters, which I didn't realise was the staff kitchen until that same night suddenly the door was closed and there was a sign on the door saying . . . out of bounds to parents—you have got to use the parents room . . . well that was a bit of a shock because there I had been using it sort of well freely and suddenly realised that oh may be I shouldn't have been using it and may be everyone was talking about me . . . but the door had never been closed before so I hadn't seen this sign. And I didn't want to use the family room because it was filthy. (Gasquoine, 1996, p. 71)

The violence of this experience was hidden within a sign on the door. The woman had been freely using a kitchen that was simply there. The sign on the door telling her not to had a deep effect on her. She imagined the staff might be talking about her. She had used the kitchen in innocence, thinking she had every right to do so. Now she is left feeling guilty, as though she deliberately went where she was not allowed to go. To make it worse, the kitchen she is now expected to use is filthy. Nevertheless, the main thrust of this story is not about the state of the other kitchen, but the guilt she felt in disobeying the sign. It seems that no one was even aware of her disobedience, except she herself. The sense of guilt remains. An outsider reading this story is likely to be disturbed by the "power over" tactics of institutional care and the inequity in cleanliness. In the midst of such an experience, while the self may rationally perceive the power over as wrong, the experience is still one of guilt.

Feeling Used

Another example of institutional power is seen in a student's comment:

There are a few niggly things that annoy me. It's to do with the fact that I am a student and I'm not getting paid. I'm contributing to the workload and some people sit around doing nothing and they are getting paid and they know more than me. (Thompson, 2000, p. 123)

This student exposes the frustration that is the aftermath of the everyday violence of "feeling used." In his disempowered status of student, others expect him to do the work while they do nothing. There is a real sense of injustice for him because they are paid to do the work and he is not. The violence of injustice stays with him as annoyance. From the student's perspective, it is not right, but there is little that he can do about it. From a broader perspective, one could argue that the practitioners are giving the student the gift of experiencing a workload. They may not interpret his frustration as "violence" but as necessary training ground. Who, then, determines when an experience that is perceived as violent is nevertheless justified?

Everyday violence lives in everyday experience. The violencing experience brings the person to a mood, which lingers, dominates, niggles, or, as in the shower story, may bring forth tears. The mood comes again at the thought of another encounter. The violence of everyday is not confined to a day but rather lives in the everyness of experience. Whether or not there is an explanation for the violence is irrelevant to the people experiencing the violence, unless perhaps their feelings are recognized and the explanation is offered to dispel misconceptions and to offer apology.

Everyday Violence, Everyday

Finally, here is a long story of a woman's experience in the days following the birth of her first child. The violence of her experience is not only in the everydayness but also in the every day:

The day after the birth I felt alone in that big place bustling with people. The midwife, who I thought would be in the first night to help me, showed up at about 5 o'clock and said, "Hi, how are you?" I thought, "Oh God, wow, at last, she has arrived. I can talk, I can find out things and ask her everything." And it was like, "How are you? Fine. Right. Well. I have to go. Don't want to get caught in the traffic." In and out in a minute.

I assume when you are in hospital, because you have an independent midwife, they don't really allocate you a midwife. My midwife never came again, I never saw her again. So she deserted me, and I wasn't really getting . . . well . . . I'm not one to ask, not one to push the bell. Perhaps I should have pushed the bell a bit more. I felt lost and alone.

They tried to help with breastfeeding, but he didn't latch on, and they tried, but they just, you know, taking this very bruised little head and whacking it against my breast. Then he would get upset, and they would stop and put him back in his crib. They just weren't there. I felt rejected.

They mentioned I should try to express. That was another thing perhaps I should have read up on. I can see some of it was my fault because I should have read about it more at the time, but you don't really think you need to because you think, "everyone is there, staff will be there," but I think I didn't have any one. I didn't feel like anyone was particularly interested. Finally a nurse gave me a nipple shield to help with latching on. She helped me with that, and he did seem to be latching on, he did seem to be getting something. And sort of the advice, "Oh, try to wean him off later on." And so this solved the immediate problem, he seemed to be getting something, and his weight wasn't dropping. He put on a little bit to go home.

Even right from the word go I wasn't feeding him enough, but I didn't know that. It was normal for him to be upset at that time of the night, and I had fed him before, why try again now? I had just fed him. I think right back then he was trying to tell me he was hungry, but oh no, it will come, and so I came home.

I had this sort of thing, well you feed new babies sort of 4 hourly or when they ask, you know, on demand. He just didn't demand that. He slept so much. He would fall asleep on the breast, and fall asleep for ages . . . that is what babies do. And then, of course, my midwife couldn't come to see me and sent someone else who came. She was ok, but. . . . She arrived, and she tried to give him some. She gave some more suggestions about the nipple shield and tried to cut it down. But the whole time, nobody watched me feed. Nobody sat, I know it is pretty boring, but nobody sat and watched what I was doing for a feed. Then she said, "When do you want me to come again?" She must have felt I was confident, "she obviously thinks she doesn't need to come every day" "the original midwife wants to come, but she can't come today" . . . I was finding it was quite a sort of gap. I think it was only 4 days, but at this stage it did count.

Finally the original midwife came to see how I was getting on, took one look at the baby, weighed him, and said, "My God, you have to get some food into this baby." He was very scrawny, and there were spots and things, well, you didn't know what to expect. They asked the question, "Are the nappies

wet?" but not "how wet?" I had no idea they were supposed to be that wet.
"They are wet, yes" but not "how wet." I did say, "They would have a little spot
here, you know, orangey as though he was dehydrated." She said, "Well they
get that after they are born," but this is about a week now, over a week, and
still to be having that. It had been left so long until we finally realised. When
the original one finally came back and weighed the baby, he had lost so much
weight. He had just been really dehydrated. (Smythe, 1998, pp. 195–197)

This woman wept as she told me of this experience, which had happened many months previously. It had been hugely traumatic in her life
at the time, and it seemed that the memories of it continued to haunt
her, especially as she contemplated the thought of having a second child.

The violence in this story is perhaps akin to the indifferent and ne-
glectful modes of care described by Heidegger (1995). It seems that
while these midwives went through the motions of providing care, they
were not being caring. They did not stop and ask, they did not stop and
watch, and they appeared not to stop and think. Perhaps most telling
is that they did not stop to "be there." They flew in and out, giving no
time. This woman and her baby needed time. They needed the time to
find out how, to talk about concerns, to be checked. All the midwife
saw as she rushed in and out was a semblance of a new mother "coping."
That is not how it was at all, yet the mother felt unable to reveal her
real needs for she knew she was expected to cope. When finally the
midwife weighed the baby, it seems she puts the blame for his dehydration on this mother who had been trying so hard to do her best. She
now not only experiences the violence of being "uncared for" but now
the added violence of having to take the blame. On top of that is her
huge concern about her baby.

This story makes me angry. Why was this woman exposed to so much
violence at such a vulnerable period of her motherhood? Yet at the same
time, I imagine if a complaint was made against this midwife, she would
defend her practice as being safe and appropriate. She would say she
visited regularly, asked the woman when she needed her to come, identified the dehydration, dealt with it. She would say she had done what
was expected of her. The tasks would be ticked off. The notion of violence would be far from her mind.

Yet, perhaps there is another side to this story. Maybe the midwife
was trapped in the cycle of too many births, not enough sleep, too many
"problems" of care, not enough time. The practitioner cannot be di-

vorced from her own world, where she may be being stretched in many different directions, with each woman wanting to feel cared for. It is a tension of the hermeneutic circle of parts and whole (Gadamer, 1982) where the client represents but one part of the practitioner's world. To understand the violence there is a need to understand the whole, yet the whole cannot exist without the component parts. One must not forget, however, that the "part" in this story is a vulnerable mother and baby. Can the violence of being uncared for ever be acceptable, even in the light of the big picture?

How Has the Violence of Everyday Practice Been Revealed?

This gathering of data suggests that people, be they clients, students, or practitioners, experience violence that is unintentional and unrecognized and therefore goes by without thought. Yet, the experience of the "self" reveals both the act of violence and the ongoing lingerings that follow the experience. It seems that violence happens when the "other" is not in attunement with the mood and, therefore, the need of the other. The attunement needs time and willingness. The person-to-person relationship has potential for violence in every encounter. It seems that the violence is more likely to be experienced when the self is distracted by the expectations of the institution and therefore does not notice, or is not able to respond, to the calling of the moment of "now" for that person, in that situation, feeling (possibly in a manner that is hidden) however he or she feels. Violence is not restricted to health practitioners' effects on clients but is also shown in the response of practitioners to the demands put on them by clients. Yet, amidst the stories of violence are images of hope caught in the sharing of tears and in the hard-won respect.

Violence was deliberately sought out and uncovered for the purpose of this analysis. There needs to be a remembering that, for the most part, violence is hidden and unnoticed. The question that calls from this study is "where is the violence in our own practice that we are not yet aware of?" I suggest this is not a question that we can ever answer for ourselves. It will only be when we ask the people we interact with how they experience our relationship that we will begin to understand how violence might be the consequence of our everyday actions. Perhaps research can hint at what we need to be mindful of, but research is not the thing in itself. Each one of us must take on the responsibility for our own being-with-others.

This opens up the question "who is other?" Lévinas (1984), a philosopher influenced by Heidegger, offers his interpretation of other, which takes us back to the self. Other can only be encountered in a face-to-face relationship where self is one of the faces. The other "'regards' me, not in order to "perceive" me, but in "concerning me," in "mattering to me as someone for whom I am answerable." The other, who—in this sense—regards me, is the face (Lévinas, 1995, p. 124). It is in this answerability that Lévinas suggests we find our individuality and "agree to depose or dethrone myself—to abdicate my position of centrality—in favour of the vulnerable other" (1984, p. 63). He cites the quote from Dostoyevsky: "We are all responsible for everyone else—but I am more responsible than all the others" (1984, p. 67). He describes such responsibility as inexhaustible "for with the other our accounts are never settled" (1995, p. 125). Such an understanding of other is much more than a recognition of difference. It is a call, a demand, an ethical charge that I will be concerned for the other, even more so than I am concerned for myself. Self and other are not two separate people whose paths happen to cross. In the crossing, other calls to self, even in the not calling. Lévinas suggests: "I can never escape the fact that the other has demanded a response from me *before* I affirm my freedom to respond to his demand" (1984, p. 63). This study has revealed that the demanded response of the other often goes by unheeded. The other makes the call, but the self, in a world of institutional demands, has become very practiced at not hearing that call. Perhaps, in fairness, the call of the "they" (Heidegger, 1995) has become louder and more dominant. The practitioner may experience the tension of the call of the face before her and the demand of the rules, the busyness, the expectations. Yet, it seems in this study that practitioners often did not recognize a demand from the face in front of them. Perhaps it was the practitioner who provoked the experience that brought forth the demand, by which stage the practitioner had turned away and did not see. Perhaps practitioners neglect to stop and look into the face of the other, to see the pleading of the eyes. Or perhaps practitioners have come to understand that they do not have enough time, energy, or courage to break out of the routine, task-focused behavior by which their practice is measured. Violence is pervasive as well. The nurse does not see the pleading in the patient's eyes, nor does the patient see the pressure upon the nurse. Perhaps the nurse does not ask certain questions because priorities of care dictate but vows to get back to these concerns tomorrow. In a system designed to be efficient and cost effective, perhaps the violence is perpetuated. Can nurses be critiqued for violence of everyday practice without simultaneously critiquing the system in which they work, a system that refuses to pay for the healthcare everyone dreams about? Is it time to abandon this system?

The call to address the violence of everyday practice comes not just from the realization that it happens, but also that its consequences live on. The occupational therapy client waits in dread for the next visit. The tension stayed with the patient in pain all day long. The woman who innocently used the wrong kitchen is encompassed by guilt. The woman who experienced day after day of violence weeps at the memories of the awfulness of that experience. This is the call of being, of what is ownmost to experience, of how the experience felt and continues to feel. This study asks the reader to hear the call. It is an echo of the calls: "We are called to care for one another and to be with others as we would like them to be with us" (Lashley, Neal, Slunt, Berman, & Hultgren, 1994, p. 207). I argue, however, that it is often not that the person does not want to care, but that the systems of practice have stripped the word care of its meaning. In a climate of economic rationalism, doing will always take precedence over caring, for doing brings measurable outputs. Perhaps it is the responsibility of researchers to bring to the light the consequences of care that is not caring.

How Can It Be That Violence Exists in Our Being-With-Others?

It could be argued that healthcare practitioners, by the very nature of their work, heed the call to care. How is it that such people, who are engaged in "being caring" can have the effect of being violent without even knowing? What is robbing "being" of its drive to be "concerned for?" Heidegger (1999) wrote in the 1930s of his perceptions of the three influences that were the cause of the abandonment of being: calculation, acceleration, and the outbreak of massiveness. I bring my interpretation of these to this discussion to see if they resonate with the world 60 years on.

Calculation describes a world that has been taken over by guiding principles and rules that imply the certainty of plans. Everything must be adjusted to the laid-down expectations. In such a world Heidegger (1999) warns us "there is no longer need for the question concerning what is ownmost to truth" (p. 84). Recall the stories of the mother and child admitted to a ward where they didn't belong, the reflections on the system of care that someone with a miscarriage must go through, the order to bottle feed. All of these are examples of practitioners caught up in predetermined plans and systems. The violence emerged when they forgot to stop and question what was "ownmost to truth." The mother knew her son simply needed care, the ward was irrelevant. The obstetrician knew that the system was creating violence in the care his clients received. The breastfeeding mother knew there was a truth beyond the preplanned decision of the medical staff. It seems that when truth becomes locked into predetermined calculations there is risk of violence. Are these examples of practitioners caught up in predetermined plans and systems in which individuals are controlled and manipulated to meet an idealized norm?

Acceleration refers to the speeding up of being that has been brought about by the possibilities of doing things faster, for example, through the use of technology. Heidegger (1999) tells us this means "not-being-able-to-bear the stillness of hidden growth and awaiting" (p. 84). There are examples of acceleration in the stories. There was the nurse who rushed the dressing of the man in pain, not having the time to wait in the stillness, to find the way that would help him to be with the pain. There was the nurse who said she would come back to help with the bath and didn't, perhaps because she was caught up in the fastness of the world around her. There were the two doctors involved in the care of the woman having the miscarriage who tried to engage her in a counseling relationship while she was enduring the pain and the trauma of the experience. In the acceleration, are we encouraged to multitask rather than take the time to do things in their own time? In the era of economic rationalism (Lawler, 1997) time is money, therefore time is budgeted and rationalized. Heidegger reminds us of the danger of controlling time at the expense of "being." When there is no time, or not enough time, then there are possibilities of violence. Is it acceptable to use lack of time as an excuse for violence, or is it time to refocus on priorities?

The outbreak of massiveness refers to the gathering of the many and the all, who are known as what "towers over them" (Heidegger, 1999, p. 85). Through such networks of communication, Heidegger tells us that "what is not ownmost . . . spreads" (p. 85). Amongst the massiveness, the rare and unique (where being is found in its ownmost) is abandoned. This could be likened to the professional body of knowledge, the research findings, and the standards of practice that dictate how practice should be at a local, national, and, indeed in today's world, global level. Amidst such massiveness, the experience of the individual gets lost. Recall the doctors who asked their list of assessment questions, the midwife who visited the breastfeeding mother to do the tasks, and the women who kept ringing the midwife at her home. None of these behaviors were about individuals deciding for themselves in relation to a specific situation. They were rather about the individuals being caught up in their understandings of "this is what I am expected to do." The massiveness creates predetermined ways of being that take away from the being itself. The ownmost, what is there, what is happening, what it feels like, is disregarded. The voice of the massiveness is much louder, much more strident, much harder to ignore, yet much more likely to cause violence. To dwell in the ownmost requires us to listen to the stillness from where we will hear the hesitant whisper.

Heidegger (1999) goes on to suggest that accompanying these three influences is "divesting, publicizing and vulgarizing of all attunement" (p. 86). He talks of a world that has become artificial in its attitudes and where the meaning of words has been lost, to become only a shell. The "all gathering of a possible mindfulness is removed and mindfulness itself is scorned as something strange and weak" (p. 86). Often in the interpretation of the stories I came to see a lack of mindfulness, no thought of what the consequences might be for the other. Often it was apparent that the people causing the violence had no insight into the harm they were inflicting. If only the midwife had been mindful of the effect of her words "failed homebirth," if only the supervisor had been mindful of what it might be like to be a student giving a patient a barium enema without having ever seen one before, if only the doctors had recognized that it was important to the mother that they saw her little son as a person. There were examples of violence in every story. Mindfulness may have seen what was in the face of the other and may have forestalled the violence.

Heidegger (1999) suggests that "all of these signs of abandonment of being point to the beginning of the *epoch of total lack of questioning of all things and of all machinations*" (p. 86). I would suggest that the world of healthcare has been overrun with "machinations." At every turn there is policy, protocol, evidence-based practice, theories of practice, professional guidelines, codes of ethics, textbooks, and editorial standards. Upholding and confirming these machinations are the ever-increasing threats of litigation (Flint, 1997; Ranjan, 1993; Symonds, 1993). The machinations are established and holding strong. Nevertheless, the challenge Heidegger presents is also enabling. Through the insights he offers, we can make our own interpretation of the meanings embedded in healthcare. Each person must question the dictates on his or her practice and bring those questions to the wider forum. And in the moment of practice itself, each person must again question the "how" of his or her practice. Practitioners need to seek the ownmost, the experience in itself. They/we are called to have the courage to move beyond the machinations to what calls us in the being. The call will be found in the face of other, if only we take the time to look and to see and to hear.

Conclusion

Heidegger (1999) tells us that "in the epoch of total lack of questioning 'problems' *will* pile up and rush around" (p. 86). This study has uncovered a pile of those problems that are rushing around in the world of everyday practice. I do not pretend that there are any easy solutions. The world of calculation, acceleration, and massiveness will not retreat at our bidding. Nevertheless, there is nothing stopping each one of us from being mindful, from asking questions, or from looking directly into the face of the other. The woman, in recounting her story of the shower, said "I actually needed a bit more 'being with' than I got." That was all she was asking for, being with.

At the close of this study I am drawn back to the quote of Caussin (OED, 1970, p. 222): "The most Sacred things are violenced, and the most Profane are licenced." This study has revealed the licensing of the habits and rituals of practice that get the job done. To follow the imposed expectations calls for duty and obedience. The actions of the licensed behaviors are observed, judged, and deemed appropriate. Meanwhile, hidden and silent, the sacred is violenced. The sacred self is ignored, neglected, or assumed. The face that would reveal the sacred becomes a blur, a face among many. The violence of the everyday, with no thought, tramples on the self, wounding and scarring. The reminder comes from Lévinas (1984) that we are all responsible, and each one of us is more responsible than everyone else. Therein lies the hope.

Violencing
client as self is
waiting, expecting, hoping
practitioner as other is
caring, helping, trying
they come together
it happens.
the other walks off,
not noticing
the self stays
smarting, wounded, confused
not understanding
experiencing the violence.
it comes from nowhere
so unexpectedly, so undeservedly.
it is not about 'what was'
but 'what was not'
in the 'being of the everyday'
the face is not drawn to face
the mindfulness is absent
the questions stay silent
and the sacred is violenced. [italics added]

Acknowledgments: I thank Nancy Diekelmann for encouraging me a second time to conceive the idea of such a paper. I acknowledge the generous support of the people whose studies were gathered together to enable the birthing of this paper. I further acknowledge the guidance of Deb Spence and the Publication Action Group of AUT in the laboring of the paper, and the reviewers in bringing it to birth.

References

Benner, P., Tanner, C., & Chesla, C. (1996). *Expertise in nursing practice*. New York: Springer.

Castellani, B., & Wear, D. (2000). Physicians views of practising professionalism in the corporate age. *Qualitative Health Research, 10*, 490–506.

Doncliff, B. (2000). Making nursing visible and valuable. *Kai Tiaki, Nursing New Zealand, 6*(11), 24–25.

Flint, C. (1997). Midwives *will* carry the can. *Midwives, 110*(1311), 96.

Gadamer, H. G. (1982). *Truth and method* (G. Barden & J. Cumming, Trans.). New York: Crossroads. (Original work published 1960)

Gasquoine, S. (1996). *Constant Vigilance. The lived experience of mothering a hospitalised child*. Unpublished master's thesis, Massey University, Palmerston North, New Zealand.

Grondin, J. (1995). *Sources of hermeneutics*. Albany: State University of New York Press.

Heidegger, M. (1995). *Being and time* (J. Macquarrie & E. Robinson, Trans.). Oxford, England: Basil Blackwell. (Original work published 1927)

Heidegger, M. (1999). *Contributions to philosophy (from enowning)* (P. Emad & K. Maly, Trans.). Bloomington: Indiana University Press. (Original work published 1989)

Kaelin, E. F. (1989). *Heidegger's being and time. A reader for readers*. Gainesville: Florida State University Press.

Kahn, D. (1999). Making the best of it: Adapting to the ambivalence of a nursing home, *Qualitative Health Research, 9*, 119–132.

King, M. (1964). *Heidegger's philosophy, a guide to his basic thought*. Oxford, England: Basil Blackwell.

Lashley, M., Neal, M., Slunt, E., Berman, L., & Hultgren, F. (1994). *Being called to care*. Albany: State University of New York Press.

Lawler, J. (1997). Knowing the body and embodiment: Methodologies, discourses and nursing. In J. Lawler (Ed), *The body in nursing*. South Melbourne, Australia: Churchill Livingstone.

Lawler, J. (1998). Phenomenologies as research methodologies for nursing: From philosophy to researching practice. *Nursing Inquiry, 5*, 104–111.

Lévinas, E. (1984). Emmanuel Lévinas. In R. Kearney (Ed.), *Dialogues with contemporary continental thinkers* (pp. 47–70). Manchester, England: University Press.

Lévinas, E. (1995). *Outside the subject*. (W. B. Smith, Trans.). London: The Athlone Press. (Original work published 1993)

Madjar, I. (1998). *Giving comfort and inflicting pain*. Edmonton, Canada: Qualitative Institute Press.

The National Health Committee (1999). *Review of maternity services in New Zealand*. Wellington, New Zealand: National Health Committee.

Opie, A. (1998). "Nobody's asked me for my view:" Users' empowerment by multidisciplinary health teams. *Qualitative Health Research, 8*, 188–206.

The Oxford English Dictionary (Vol. 12). (1970). Oxford, England: Clarendon Press.

Paddy, A. (2000). *Experiencing the relationship: The client and the community occupational therapist. A phenomenological study*. Unpublished master's thesis, Auckland University of Technology, Auckland, New Zealand.

Ranjan, V. (1993). Obstetrics and the fear of litigation. *MIDIRS Midwifery Digest, 3,* 360–362.

Savage, J. (2000). One voice, different tunes: Issues raised by dual analysis of a segment of qualitative data. *Journal of Advanced Nursing, 31,* 1493–1500.

Smith, L., & Daughtrey, H. (2000). Weaving the seamless web of care: An analysis of parents' perceptions of their needs following discharge of their child from hospital. *Journal of Advanced Nursing, 31,* 812–820.

Smythe, E. (1998). *'Being safe' in childbirth. A hermeneutic interpretation of the narratives of women and practitioners.* Unpublished doctoral thesis, Massey University, Palmerston North, New Zealand.

Soderberg, S., Lundman, B., & Norberg, A. (1999). Struggling for dignity: The meaning of women's experience of living with fibromyalgia. *Qualitative Health Research, 9,* 575–587.

Spence, D. (1999). *Prejudice, paradox and possibilities: Nursing people from cultures other than one's own.* Unpublished doctoral thesis, Massey University, Palmerston North, New Zealand.

Sykes, J. B. (1985). *The concise Oxford dictionary of current English.* Oxford, England: Clarendon Press.

Symonds, E. (1993). Litigation and the cardiotocogram. *British Journal of Obstetrics and Gynaecology, 100*(9), 8–9.

Thompson, A. (1999). *'Showing the way'. The meaning of supervision and learning for student diagnostic medical radiation technologists and their supervisors.* Unpublished master's thesis, Auckland University of Technology, Auckland, New Zealand.

Van Manen, M. (1990). *Researching lived experience.* London, Ontario: The Althouse Press.

Weiss, J., & Hutchinson, S. (2000). Warnings about vulnerability in clients with diabetes and hypertension. *Qualitative Health Research, 10,* 521–537.

5

Telling Stories of Suffering and Survival

Women and Violence

Claire Burke Draucker and Joanne M. Hessmiller

A life becomes meaningful when one sees himself or herself as an actor within the context of a story, be it a cultural tale, a religious narrative, a family saga, the march of science, a political movement, and so forth.

G. S. Howard, "Culture Tales"

Introduction

Interpretive researchers often use narratives, stories people tell about their lives, as the primary source of "data" for their inquiry. Most investigators, however, are concerned with the content of the stories rather than with how and why the stories are told. Researchers seldom reflect on the strategies participants use for storytelling or consider the meaning of the structure of their narratives. Many analytic approaches are designed to code, summarize, or organize the participants' words in a conceptual schemata, with the goal of achieving a "higher" level of abstraction or producing theory. By failing to attend to the "narrative character of the talk" (Chase, 1995, p. 1), researchers may miss the opportunity to appreciate how individuals make sense of the life experiences that are the focus of study.

In this chapter we (Claire and Joanne) explore the narrative character of the talk of women who tell stories about their experiences of violence.

204

Claire is a psychologist and psychiatric mental health nurse who specializes in counseling women who have been sexually abused as children or who experience intimate violence later in life. Joanne is a social worker who has worked in the Battered Woman's Movement in the United States for the past 20 years and focuses her clinical work and research on the prevention of intimate violence. We both have studied women's experiences of violence in qualitative studies, and our findings have been presented in various venues (Draucker, 1992, 1999; Draucker & Madsen, 1999; Draucker & Stern, 2000; Hessmiller, 1998). We met at the Advanced Institute for Heideggerian Hermeneutics, held annually at the University of Wisconsin–Madison. In addition to sharing an interest in the same content area—violence against women—and in the same research approach—interpretive phenomenology—we discovered that we had made similar observations about the stories we were hearing from women who had experienced violence; that is, we had unearthed consistencies in *how* women told stories of violence and concluded that these "ways of telling" might reveal something significant about women's experiences.

Joanne, for example, in her study of the meaning that battered women make of their experiences, found that each woman told her story in essentially the same way, with absolutely no prompting from Joanne and without contact with one another. Each women spontaneously told the story of the "first time" and the "worst time" they were abused. This observation both fascinated and perplexed Joanne, leading her to wonder what the form of these stories might be saying about the experience of women in this culture.

Claire was particularly struck by the narrative of Sarah (pseudonym), a 24-year-old Caucasian college student who had participated in Claire's grounded theory study of women's responses to sexual assault by male intimates (Draucker & Stern, 2000). Sarah had experienced four date–acquaintance rapes since the age of 17. Although most of the interviews conducted by Claire focused on how women cope following an episode of violence, Sarah's interview was clearly dedicated to describing the assault incidents themselves. She described each rape in story form, describing the assault, as well as the events leading up to and following it, in much detail. While the content of each rape story was different, Claire had observed how the structure of each story (described below) was quite similar. Claire wondered what the parallel forms of the four rape stories revealed about Sarah's experiences of violence.

Based on the assumption that examining the narrative character of stories can result in a greater appreciation and deeper understanding of life experiences, we decided to focus on the practices of storytelling and explore what might be revealed by the form and structure of women's stories of violence. Lieblich, Tuval-Mashiach, & Zilber (1998) distinguished studies that are content oriented, in which narratives are used for the investigation of a research question, from studies that are form oriented, in which the narratives themselves are the research object. Content-oriented studies are concerned with the explicit content of the participants' stories, such as the who, what, when, and why, or the implicit content of the story, such as the motivations of the characters or the meaning of symbolic imagery. In contrast, a form-oriented approach is concerned with the formal aspects of the stories, such as the narrative style, plot structure, linguistic style, sequence of events, and use of metaphors. We agree with Lieblich and colleagues that "formal aspects of structure, as much as content, express the identity, perceptions, and values of the storyteller . . . [and that] analyzing the structure of the story will therefore reveal the individual's personal construction of his or her evolving life experience" (p. 88).

We begin by first considering the function of storytelling, especially for those who have suffered, and then by examining the structure and form of Sarah's four rape stories using three analytic strategies discussed by Antaki (1994). We chose Sarah's text for our first attempt at narrative analysis because (a) she spent most of the interview describing the rapes themselves, in story form, rather than discussing how she had coped following the violence; (b) her interview contained four discrete, but clearly interrelated, stories of sexual assault that seemed parallel in form; and (c) in addition to describing the four rapes, she provided much additional information about her family and her childhood, thereby providing the historical context to her sexual assault stories.

Antaki (1994) argued that storied accounts of life events serve to construct social realities. Examining the structure of everyday first-person accounts may reveal how the account achieves its meaning. Formal descriptions of accounts draw from literary stylistics, which is the study of how the formal features of a text influences interpretation. While some literary analysis may focus on cognitive structures that create narrative coherence, Antaki is interested primarily in culturally determined rules for the performance of practical storytelling.

The first approach to narrative analysis that we used to examine the structure of Sarah's rape stories is based on the assumption that narratives reflect a rule-bound sequence of steps. The steps of an account are examined for function, that is, what the parts "do" to get the story told, rather than categorical content. Narratives are pared down to a basic sequencing. The core narrative, thought to capture the life experiences, or the social identity, of the participants, is identified. We therefore pared down each of Sarah's four rape stories to a basic sequencing of events, identified a core narrative, and speculated on what the core narrative might reveal about Sarah's experiences.

Second, we considered how sociocultural factors influenced the formal aspects of Sarah's storytelling. Antaki (1994) argued that narratives are infused with background beliefs that remain unarticulated; all narratives are circumscribed by cultural expectations of "proper sequential unfolding" (Antaki, 1994, p. 100). A cultural interpretation of a narrative is "an interpretation of how [the stories] express and reflect broader cultural frameworks of meaning" (Mishler, 1986, p. 244). Mishler stressed that such interpretation requires an understanding of the local and general circumstances of the participants.

Antaki (1994) proposed that one may also analyze storied accounts by comparing them to classic literary forms or existing classifications of types of narratives. This approach is based on the assumption that people explain themselves by "invoking stylistically well-known story types" (p. 96). We conclude our analysis by considering whether Sarah's story resembles any classic story types by determining whether Sarah's stories fit into existing typologies of illness–trauma stories.

Sarah's Story

Sarah was a 24-year-old Caucasian college student majoring in dance who had participated in an unstructured interview for a study Claire had conducted on women's responses to sexual violence by male intimates (Draucker & Stern, 2000). Prior to the interview, she was informed about the purpose of the research, which was "to obtain women's descriptions of their experiences with intimate sexual violence so that health professionals might be better informed when working with women who have had such experiences," and signed an informed consent form that outlined the risks and benefits of participation. In addition, Sarah had been assured that her identity would be protected in all publications and presentations, and, therefore, her name, the names of other individuals mentioned in her narrative, and some identifying data have been changed to ensure confidentiality.

Sarah had experienced four date–acquaintance rapes as well as several other incidents in which she was maltreated or abused by men whom she knew. She described each rape in story form. Each story included a discussion of a situation that opened up the possibility for the rape to occur (the initial condition), a series of interactions leading up to the rape, a detailed description of the rape itself, and a series of interactions following the rape.

The Core Narratives

The events of each of the four rape episodes, as described by Sarah, are presented below. The "plot" of each rape story is divided into the initial condition, events leading up to the rape, the rape, and events following the rape.

The First Rape

This first rape occurred when Sarah was almost 17. Sarah identified the characteristics of the three main individuals in her rape narrative. She described herself at the time as "a little Gothic girl, pale you know, wore everything up to the throat, the wrists, you know, wore oversized everything." She described her girlfriend, Lily, as "basically the high school slut. She was a nice girl, very, she was very loud and very obnoxious and she was like very comical and really funny and very outgoing and she was like a tomboy. . . . She slept around a lot." She stated that John, the rapist, was "this big football player guy that, you know, [was] used to women hanging all over him."

Initial Condition   When Sarah began the story of the first rape with the following description of a conversation between her and a friend, it was unclear how the conversation was related to the rape, but this did become apparent at the end of the story.

And the one night me and her [Lily], she asked me how many guys I slept with, and I said, "Only one and I'm sleeping with this guy that I'm with" and she thought that was really weird. She's like, "Nobody does, everybody else has had a lot," and I was like, you know, "I've been with him."

Before the Rape   Sarah and Lily (Sarah's friend) go to MacDonald's. Lily runs into an old boyfriend (Sam) whom her parents do not allow her to see.

Lily and Sarah plan to go to the movies; Lily asks Sarah if it's okay if Sam comes along.

Sam asks if he can bring a friend (John).

Lily arranges for John to pick them up because she cannot go out with Sam.

John shows up, meets Lily's father, and the three drive away.

When they are out of sight, Sam gets in the car. They switch seats so that Sarah is with John and Lily is with Sam. (Sarah realizes she is "set up" for a double date.)

They park in a deserted playground. John, Lily, and Sam begin to drink.

They drive to the movies. Lily and Sam stay in the car. John and Sarah go in and decide there is nothing playing they want to see.

They all go back to the playground. John and Sarah are "kicked out" of the car so Lily and Sam can be alone.

Sarah and John go to the swings.

The Rape   John begins to asks Sarah questions (e.g., what kind of music she likes).

He grabs her leg, starts to kiss her.

[She interrupts the story to explain that she later found out he had been doing drugs for 3 days.]

Sarah tries to get John "off" her and attempts to walk away. He grabs her, begins to slap her, and calls her a "tease."

He gets her tights off and asks if she wants him to put on a condom.

She screams "no" to make him stop; he says "okay—no condom" and penetrates her.

She fights and scratches. He cannot have an orgasm.

He demands oral sex; she complies but "gnaws" on his penis.

He pins her arms over her head. She continues to fight; he continues to hit her, pulling out chunks of her hair.

He continues to try to penetrate her; she resists by "flipping over."

He cuts her vagina with a pocketknife and scratches the inside of her for "punishment."

He eventually gives up; she rolls up in a ball.

After the Rape   Lily and Sam return. Sam realizes what happened and "beats up" John, forcing him to apologize to Sarah.

Lily doesn't realize what happened. She asks Sarah, "Isn't it great being a slut?"

John drives them home. Lily and Sam put Sarah in the front seat with John.

They drop Sarah off at a friend's house; she stays for the night.

She takes a bath and goes home the next day.

She bleeds for three days and stays in her room. (Sarah keeps wondering if she did anything wrong.)

[She interrupts the story to tell about her then-current boyfriend and how he controlled her dress to explain why she was dressed very conservatively the night of the rape.]

A couple of days later, she talks to Lily and discovers that Lily had told John that Sarah was a "tease" and would play hard to get but would "get into it." Lily stated she did this because she thought it was unusual that Sarah had only slept with one person.

Sarah goes to stay with her friend Jerry. She lays on his couch staring into space.

He watches over her, continually asking her if she is okay. She tells him about the rape.

He invites her to a band camp to get her mind off the rape.

The Second Rape

At camp, Jerry at first stays close to Sarah but eventually begins to spend time with other friends. Sarah meets Alex. They become friends and keep in touch with letters after the camp is over. Alex attacks Sarah twice; she tells the story of an attempted rape and an actual rape. Sarah described Alex as: "A very nice, sweet boy. Wanted to go into the Navy. Wasn't my type."

Initial Condition

I just broke up with the guy I was with. I started seeing this other guy, and he was older again and I wanted, my parents were really big on I had to go to the prom. I was not into that kind of stuff, but it made my mother happy. . . . Jake [Sarah's boyfriend] said he was going to go with me and then we broke up like a couple of days prior and then he was still going to go to the prom with me until like the day before the prom. And he gave me a call and he was like, "I am not going with you. . . ." I knew Alex had bought himself a suit for the prom, and so I gave Alex a call and I said, "Will you go to the prom with me? I know you have the suit and Jake backed out. Will you go with me?" and he's like, "Okay."

Sarah and Alex go to the prom "as friends."

He dances too close; she wonders if he's thinking this is a "real date."

They hang out with other friends, not spending much time together at the prom.

Sarah has a party after the prom. She falls asleep on the couch and wakes up to find Alex on top of her, trying to "fool around."

She pushes him off and yells at him.

Alex apologizes; he states he doesn't know why he did it.

She takes Alex home; they stop and have coffee; she is "nasty" to him.

He apologizes. They go back to being friends.

Before the Rape   In a couple of months, Sarah and Jerry go to visit Alex.

Alex asks Sarah out and she accepts.

They go to the movies, but there is "nothing good playing."

They go around his hometown looking at the local scenery.

They go to a secluded spot along a ravine.

The Rape   While they are sitting and talking at the ravine, Alex asks Sarah if he may kiss her.

She says yes and experiences the kissing as "nice."

He puts his hands up her shirt.

He lays her back on the car seat and "tries things."

She agrees to kissing and touching with her clothes on.

Without Sarah realizing it, he undoes his pants, adjusts her underwear, and penetrates her.

She pushes him off and screams at him. She leaves him at the ravine.

After the Rape   She tells Jerry and Jerry states he will never see Alex again, but Sarah asks Jerry not to get in the "middle of it."

A few days later, she goes to Jack, an old classmate and her best friend, for comfort.

The Third Rape

Sarah describes Jack as "a very good looking guy and all the girls were chasing after him, and I mean every girl in my high school wanted to go out with him. It was just disgusting, and he was dating everybody and everything, and Jack was like a little bit strange."

Initial Condition

At the time, I was going through therapy for depression and eating disorder, and my therapist kept telling me to talk about things and let things out that way and it was working, you know. I had to vent it out and I had no one to turn to and I didn't really want to upset my girlfriends by going to them with it. And, like, at the time I was like still like confused and the rest of my girlfriends were, you know, "you were easy."

Before the Rape   Jack invites her over. She tells him she wants to talk about the rape.

They sit on his porch and have a soda.

She tells him about the rape.

He is sympathetic ("that's really shitty").

Sarah calms down; she feels happy.

She and Jack go inside and move to his bed to talk because Jack has no living room.

The Rape   Jack asks Sarah why she likes James (mutual friend) better than him.

Sarah explains James protects her—never "tries" anything.

Tells Jack she is not attracted to him, she feels like he's a brother.

He grabs her and kisses her.

Sarah protests, "What about Jennifer?" (Jack's girlfriend).

He bites her throat in a "joking" manner.

She tells him to back off.

Jack starts to get aggressive.

She wants him to hold her.

He keeps touching her; she again tries to push him off.

He "shifts things around," he quickly penetrates her and has an orgasm.

Sarah crawls backward, yells "Get the fuck off me," and asks him why he did that.

He tells her she needed to be calmed down because she was mixed up about sex.

After the Rape   Sarah tells her cousin, who says Jack took advantage of her vulnerability and confusion.

She stays upset with Jack for 2 months. Sarah tells his girlfriend about the rape, and the girlfriend breaks up with Jack.

She later runs into a girl who had dated Jack; the girl reveals Jack had also raped her.

The Fourth Rape

Sarah goes away to college and meets Hank. He asks her to go to the mall, but she is hesitant. She now does not like to go places with men alone.

Initial Condition

The girls [in her dorm, who knew Hank] said, "He's [Hank] real nice. He's like a really great friend and everything." And he was friends with them. He had female friends. I was just like, okay, he has female friends and none of them ever said he came on to them, so I was just like okay and everything. He showed up and my one problem was, my roommate is from Morocco and she's not allowed to go anywhere without her cousin, and her cousin was going to come with us and everything and she was like waiting for her escort. And he was just like going to follow up and then take off. . . . But she ended up, he didn't show up, so she's like, "I can't go."

Before the Rape   Hank and Sarah "joke around" and get in the car.
They drive through "farmland galore."
Hank turns off the main road and turns into a "creepy" dirt road.
He stops the car, telling Sarah he just wants to talk to her.

The Rape   He starts touching her hand.
She asks if they aren't going to the mall.
She asks to go, and he asks if he can kiss her.
She says it's okay.
He kisses her and also starts to fondle her "a bit."
Sarah starts to push and move away.
He pulls the back of her hair and kisses her throat.
He puts his hand on her thigh, and she pushes it away, saying "no, no, no, no."
He demands oral sex; she says "no," and he yanks her hair and says "yes."
He undoes his belt while holding her hair.
She puts her hand on his stomach and digs her nails into his skin.
He pushes her head into his lap.
She "gnaws" on him.

He puts her other hand on his stomach so she will continue digging her nails into him.

She bites his thigh, smacks him "shitless," and says, "No, I don't want it."

After the Rape   A man comes out of the farmhouse nearby and asks if they are okay.

Sarah is about to say "no," but Hank says "yes, we're leaving" and starts up the car.

They drive back to the college in silence.

He asks if she had a good time, and she tells him he got too aggressive.

She confides in an old friend of the family, who confirms that Hank is "strange." He and his friends offer to beat up Hank, but Sarah says no, she doesn't want anyone to know what happened.

Hank continues to pursue her by leaving messages on her answering machine until she tells him to stop.

She later hears he raped a freshman but was not "charged" with it.

Some time after the rape, she sees Hank approach a "shy" girl in the college library, and Sarah loudly announces that he is a rapist.

The girl gets up and leaves. Hank swears at Sarah and walks out of the library.

The Storytelling of Those Who Have Suffered

Before we examine the structural aspects of Sarah's stories, we focus on Sarah as storyteller and consider the meaning of storytelling for those who suffer. Sarah clearly demonstrated what Mishler (1986) referred to as the impulse to narrate. Claire interviewed Sarah for over 2 hours. Her transcript consists of many pages of uninterrupted storytelling regarding the rapes themselves. Claire is aware that as an interviewer she has often been guilty of suppressing stories in the interest of gaining information to answer a specific research question (Mishler, 1986), but this did not occur to any great extent in Sarah's interview. Sarah was clearly intent on telling complete stories regarding all her rape experiences.

Coles (1989) argued that storytelling is "everyone's bedrock capacity" (p. 30); Taylor (1996) pointed out that human beings are natural and obsessive storytellers; and Bruner (1990) stressed that humans have a "readiness or predisposition to organize experience into a narrative form, into plot structures and the rest" (p. 43). Roberts (1999) stated:

Delightfully and inescapably we have story-telling brains, and in formatting and patterning the world around us we are little different from dream-time aboriginals (Chatwin, 1988), giving words and meanings to the landscape on which we shall then live. (p. 7)

Polkinghorne (1988) argued that narratives provide a framework for understanding the past and planning the future; they are our primary means of rendering life experiences meaningful. Mair (1988) stressed the essential nature of storytelling:

I want to claim much more than the comfortable platitude that stories are a good thing and should be attended to. Stories are habitations. We live in and through stories. They conjure worlds. We do not know the world other than as story world. Stories inform life. They hold us together and keep us apart. We inhabit the great stories of our culture. We live through stories. We are *lived* by the stories of our race and place. It is this enveloping and constituting function of stories that is especially important to sense more fully. (p. 127)

Merleau-Ponty (1945/1962) stressed that it is through our linguistic ability that we bring forth interpretation of our primary perceptual and emotional experiences (Polkinghorne, 1988). Through expression we draw meaning from experience. There is a raw meaning—a "wild logos"— that calls out for expression of those life experiences of which we have not spoken (Polkinghorne, 1988). Polkinghorne stated, "Life presents itself as a raw indication that needs to be finished by interpretation to make it meaningful" (p. 30).

Sarah's stories are stories of trauma. Life experiences of a traumatic nature demand thematic expression; they call forth stories (Roberts, 1999). The stories of individuals who suffer, or who experience life's hardships, are thought to share a common purpose. Roberts argued that:

Narrative responses to desperate circumstances offer a means of containing wild, threatening, and unpredictable experiences, and re-establishing some kind of order or relationship. . . . Story-making, as a life-supporting process, is a psychic resource, a defence [*sic*] against futility, emptiness, and formless terror. (p. 13)

As an example of the importance of storytelling in response to desperate circumstances, Roberts discussed the narrative activities of the Beirut hostages around 1993–1994. He quotes Terry Waite:

I soon realised that if I was to survive, it was essential to maintain a strong inner life. I needed to tell myself stories. In telling myself the story of my life I was maintaining a lifeline with reality I had known and lived. Characters from the past emerged to comfort, amuse and haunt. Time took on another meaning. That which I called "the past" was a part of me. My soul longed for harmony and rhythm . . . when I eventually emerged all I wanted was a pencil and notebook. The book was already written in my mind. One eminent reviewer described the book as being "egocentric." He quite failed to see that the writer was attempting to hang onto identity, because the threat of dissolving into madness was ever present. (p. 14)

We believe stories of violence have much in common with stories of illness. Both types of stories are born from circumstances that fundamentally challenge one's sense of security, self-identity, and life plans (Roberts, 1999, p. 14). Stories about violence and trauma, like those about illness, are narratives of interrupted lives. Both types of stories provide a common bond for those who tell them and serve to turn suffering into testimony.

Kleinman (1988) and Frank (1995) emphasized the importance of storytelling for those who are seriously ill, the "wounded storytellers." By illness, Kleinman means "the innately human experience of symptoms and suffering" (p. 3). He states:

Patients order their experiences of illness—what it means to them and to significant others—as personal narratives. The illness narrative is the story that patient tells, and significant others retell, to give coherence to distinctive events and long-term course of suffering. The plot lines, core metaphors, and rhetorical devices that structure the illness narrative are drawn from cultural and personal models for arranging experiences in meaningful ways and for effectively communicating those meanings. (p. 49)

Frank suggested that stories serve to repair the damage that illness does to one's sense of where one is and where one is going. Illness robs individuals of their life maps; it is through telling stories of their illness, and experiencing the "shared" nature of their stories, that they develop a new map.

The stories of illness are stories of interruptions (Frank, 1995). Disease is an interruption of life as planned, and living with illness involves living with interruption. The ill person is "infinitely interruptible"—of speech, sleep, and financial solvency. Those hospitalized are interrupted in sleep and routine, the structure of the medical history interrupts storytelling in favor of structure, and physical disability interrupts life's normal activities. The goal of the illness narrative is therefore paradoxical; it must restore "an order that the interruption fragmented, but it must also tell the truth that the interruptions will continue" (p. 59).

Storytelling gives voice to the body. Before the story, the body reveals the illness only through pain and other symptoms. Stories, however, are social; they are told to someone and are shaped by audience expectations. Storytelling transforms one's life by contributing to the lives of others. Frank (1995) argued that people do not tell stories to construct the maps of others, for each must do this for oneself, but to witness the reconstruction of one's own map.

Sarah's stories were of suffering; Frank and Kleinman would consider her a wounded storyteller. Clearly each assault is an interruption in her life as planned. She participates in Claire's original study to help healthcare providers help other women who had similar experiences to her own. Her stories allows us, as Frank would say, to witness the reconstruction of her life map.

Traumatized, violated, and ill individuals are often silenced, however, fearing their stories will meet with rejection and bring forth fear and shame. Their experiences remain, in Merleau-Ponty's terms, "wild logos." Individuals may tell themselves stories but believe that saying them aloud may carry great risk (Roberts, 1999). Because significant life events are concealed, the silenced storyteller remains invisible and disconnected.

Sarah discusses several instances in which she had been silenced as a storyteller. She does not tell her parents about the rapes until many years later because she believed that they "would not understand." On several occasions she tells friends or acquaintances about the violence she experienced, only to be betrayed by them. The most striking example of this betrayal is the incident in which she confides in Jack about her rape by Alex, only to be raped by Jack as well. Sarah also gives examples of times when she was silenced by professionals charged with helping her. She describes going to therapists who were "these stern older women who don't understand and, you know, [act like] 'if I have to listen to one more depression story, I'm going to choke.'"

When a previously unacknowledged experience is spoken, it can become integrated into one's life history. Harvey, Orbuch, Chwalisz, and Garwood (1991) emphasized that trauma stories are healing because they are the mechanism by which individuals form explanations or accounts of what might otherwise be an inexplicable tragedy. At the time of the interview, Claire was concerned that Sarah never really "got to" how she coped with the violence (the topic of the original study) because she provided such a lengthy description of the rape episodes themselves. In retrospect, however, it appears that Sarah told her stories (relatively uninterrupted by Claire) as a way of interpreting her own traumatic experiences. She was determined not to be silenced during this interview. Thus, as we examine the structure of Sarah's narrative, we do so with the assumption that her storytelling reflects, in some way, her quest to reestablish order following a series of experiences that threatened her security and sense of self and continually interrupted her life plans—as well as to help other girls and women who have experienced violence. Her stories do serve to turn suffering into testimony.

The Structure of Sarah's Stories

To understand what the structure of Sarah's rape narratives reveals about her experiences, we first had to consider the essential elements of the narrative by drawing from literature on narrative analysis, stories, and story-making. According to Gergen and Gergen (1986), in a narrative account, events are presented in a manner that demonstrates connectedness and coherence and provides a sense of movement and direction through time. Bruner (1990) outlined four "crucial grammatical constituents" required for a narrative to be effective:

It requires, first, a means for emphasizing human action or "agentivity"—action directed toward goals controlled by agents. It requires, secondly, that a sequential order be established and maintained—that events and states be "linearized" in a standard way. Narrative, thirdly, requires a sensitivity to what is canonical and what violates canonicality in human interaction. Finally, narrative requires something approximating a narrator's perspective: it cannot, in the jargon of narratology, be "voiceless." (p. 77)

Bell (1988) identified the basic structural elements of a story. All stories have a beginning, or orientation, that is recognized by the narrator and listener. The story may begin with an abstract, which is a brief summary of the plot, and an indication of the time, place, characters, and situation. The story line consists of linked categories, which are episodes connected to each other causally or temporally. The story reveals the sequence in which the episodes take place. The episodes are animated by narrative clauses that elaborate on the actions and give meaning to the events. The results of the action are revealed in the resolution. The story's ending, or coda, is acknowledged by both narrator and listener.

The plot is the thread that connects the elements of the story. Polkinghorne (1988) stated that:

The plot functions to transform a chronicle or listing of events into a schematic whole by highlighting and recognizing the contribution that certain events make to the development and outcome of the story. Without the recognition of significance given by the plot, each event would appear as discontinuous and separate, and its meaning would be limited to its categorical identification or its spatiotemporal location. (p. 19)

The plot reveals the historical and social context of the events and spotlights those occurrences that are novel or unexpected, thereby serving as an explanation for puzzling or unique phenomenon.

Kermode (1967) claimed that a plot offers relief from chronicity, or *chronos* (the Greek notion of clock time; that is, the meaningless succession of events between the beginning and the end) through *kairos* (the Greek notion of time redeemed). *Kairos* reflects the breaking of time into periods of significance, identified by the occurrence of a significant event. In a story, meaningful episodes occur when a significant event places the characters into positions that require decisions and action. Characters are responsible for the consequences of their choices, and their purposive actions provide a meaningful connection between the beginning and the end of the story. In the end, the infinite possibilities that existed in the beginning are worked out by the choices made by the characters.

Labov (1982) discussed the role of the reportable event in plot development, arguing that because a narrative takes up a larger portion of social time than is usually justifiable in conversation, the story must have a significant point so that at the end the "audience" does not ask "so what?" Reportable events, which are almost always unusual happenings, must therefore hold the audience's attention. The maximally reported event is the event most central to the characterization of the narrative; it is what the story is about. A story is credible only to the extent that it provides a plausible account of events leading up to this event and thus typically begins with a description of the conditions whereby the maximally reportable event came about. The notion of the reportable event is reminiscent of Bruner's (1990) argument that narratives deal with canonicality and exceptionality. Stories achieve their meaning by making deviations from the ordinary explicable, often by revealing the internal state, such as the desires and beliefs, of the protagonist.

Using concepts of narrative structure proposed by Gergen and Gergen (1996), Bruner (1990), Bell (1988), Polkinghorne (1988), Kermode (1967), and Labov (1982) we examine the four main sequential sections of Sarah's rape stories and put forth our interpretations about what the narrative structure reveals about her experiences.

Structural Analysis

Sarah's rape stories meet Gergen and Gergen's (1986) definition of a narrative. She clearly spells out how each incident "sets the stage" for the following incident, and ultimately, for the four assaults. She is diligent in telling us how old she was at the time of each rape and situates each rape within a particular life circumstance, for example, which school she was attending at the time. She consistently used time to structure and organize her narrative. She described the four rapes as they occurred chronologically and the events within each rape scenario as they occurred in time. Before beginning her story, she told me, "I've been raped four times. One was right before I turned 17. Two were when I was 18, and one was when I was 19, up until 20. . . ." The stories about the rapes connect her past, present, and future and provide us with a sense of her travels throughout young adulthood. Sarah's narrative style reflects the notion of *kairos* (Kermode, 1967); she breaks time into periods of significance identified by the occurrence of significant events—the four rapes. Each rape calls for her to make decisions and take action.

According to Polkinghorne (1988), all narrative plots highlight events that are unique or unexpected; events that, according to Bruner, "violate canonicality in human interaction" (p. 12). Labov (1982) would consider the rapes to be "reportable events" in Sarah's narrative—they are unusual happenings, and this justifies the time it takes to tell about them. She refers in passing to several other experiences during her life in which she was maltreated or abused but refers to these experiences as having "people trying stuff on me," apparently to distinguish these incidents from the "actual rape" incidents she chose to describe in detail for the study. Reportable events, because they are unusual, require an explanation. The four steps of each of Sarah's rape stories serve to provide a plausible account of the rape events.

Initial Condition

Sarah began each rape narrative by describing an "initial condition" that set the stage for the events leading to the rape. In each case, Sarah told of a situation in which she was betrayed, let down, or abandoned. Sarah felt she was "set up" for the first rape because Lily decided Sarah needed more sexual partners. Sarah's narrative regarding the second rape began with a discussion of how Jake backed out of going to the prom, prompting her to ask Alex to be his replacement. Alex first attempted to rape her the night of the prom. After the rape by Alex, she sought comfort from Jack because her therapist told her she needed "to talk about it [the rape]," and her girlfriends already thought she was "too easy." Jack then rapes her himself. She introduces the narrative of the fourth rape by explaining how she was supposed to go to the mall with her college roommate and Hank, but her roommate backed out of the outing because she did not have an escort as required by her custom. Having been reassured by other women in her dorm that Hank was a nice guy, Sarah went alone with him to the mall; on the way, he assaults her.

Labov (1982) argued that each person who tells a narrative faces the problem of where to begin. He stated, "The selection of the orientation section by the narrator is one of the crucial steps in the construction of the narrative and the theory of causality that supports it. In general, the speaker searches for the first set of general conditions whereby the question 'how did that come about?' is appropriately answered" (p. 229). What the structure of Sarah's narratives suggests is that being betrayed or abandoned—forsaken in some way—"set the stage" for the assaults. She could have begun each narrative with a description of the assault itself (e.g., "John was a blind date who raped me by the playground swings," or "Alex tried to rape me the night of my prom"), but for Sarah this would not have been the whole story. The "beginning" of each narrative occurred not when she was raped, but rather at the moment she was deceived or deserted.

Sarah's life story has a similar "orientation" to her rape narratives. She interrupted one of her rape narratives to explain:

My parents didn't really care for me, you know, because I was the odd kid that didn't talk to them and I kept my distance, and when I was little my parents were alcoholics and my dad was a workaholic so my parents had their own separate life and they ignored the children and I would run around the neighborhood and never, wouldn't come back for days. Other people would take me off my parents' [hands]. So my parents never were really, you know, very attached to me whatsoever, you know, I was sort of more of a burden, you know, at the time, when I was younger.

The orientation of each rape narrative, and of Sarah's life story, consists of incidents in which she is left alone to fend for herself. The function of these orientations seems to be to focus audience attention on the interpersonal context of the violence. Sarah's description of the initial condition creates an appreciation that her suffering stems not just from the assaults but from a primordial state of being forsaken.

Before the Rape

Before describing each rape, Sarah sets the scene with considerable detail. For each rape narrative, she outlines a series of events whereby she ended up alone with the rapist in a vulnerable position. She is raped by John after they find out there are no "good" movies playing and they are "kicked out" of the car by the other couple they were with, thereby ending up alone at the playground swings. She ends up at an isolated ravine with Alex—again after a change of plans because there were no "good" movies playing. She describes a series of events in which she and Jack move from the porch where they were talking to Jack's bed because he has no living room. She reveals how she ended up alone with Hank in a deserted area:

You know, so he picked me, you know he came over and picked me up and everything was fine. We were like joking around and everything. Got into the car. We were driving from [the college town], there's farm land galore around. There's all you see—is cornfields—and like we're driving on the road and all

I'm seeing is cornfields. I'm like, "Where is the mall?" And he's like, "It's 20 minutes outside of, you know, [the college town]. You have to go toward [the nearest large city] and everything. So it's like okay and everything. He's like, "Don't worry. We'll be driving through these little towns here and there." So I was like, "Okay."

As Labov (1982) argued, "The speaker has to find a credible way to bridge the gap between the initial conditions and the reportable event with a series of intervening actions" (p. 229). The intervening events described by Sarah bridged the gap between the orientation (the circumstances in which Sarah was forsaken) and the reportable event (the actual sexual assault). The events that Sarah tells to fill the gap reflect chance circumstances, such as what's playing at the movies, how an apartment is arranged, and the physical terrain between the college dorm and the shopping mall. Including such details in the narrative serves to focus audience attention on how "fate" played a role in the rapes. Sarah's explanation of the rapes stressed that she was alone with these men by chance, not choice.

The Rape

There were also striking similarities between the four narratives in relationship to how Sarah described each assault. For all the situations, Sarah discussed in some detail how the rapist began with kissing and noninvasive sexual activities. In two of the instances (Alex and Hank), the boy asked if he could kiss her. In all cases, the boys became increasingly aggressive despite her pleas for them to stop the sexual activity. Both Alex and Hank demanded oral sex and Sarah complied but "gnawed" on their penises. With John and Hank, she fought back physically as well as verbally. Alex and Jack penetrated her quickly, surprising her. Sarah made it very clear in each of her narratives at which point she says "no," how she tried to resist the assault, and how outraged she was when the assault was over. Her explanation of the rape emphasized that she did not desire, at any point, the invasive sexual activity.

After the Rape

Sarah's descriptions of the aftermath of the four rapes also share commonalities. Sarah reveals that after each rape she seeks solace from a friend. After the rape by John she seeks comfort and support from Jerry. He watches over her while she is at his house and invites her to camp. After her rape by Alex, she seeks comfort from Jack and at first feels understood and supported by him. After the rape by Jack, Sarah gains support from a cousin. After the rape by Hank, she talks to an old friend who validates her conclusion that Hank is "strange."

In three of the cases, she reveals how male friends or acquaintances retaliate—or volunteer to retaliate—against the rapist. Sam beats up John and makes him apologize to Sarah when Sam returns to the playground swings and realizes what John had done to Sarah. Jerry volunteers to never have contact with Alex again because Alex raped Sarah, but Sarah asks him not to get in the "middle of it." Friends offer to beat up Hank after the rape, but Sarah asks them not to because she does not want anyone to know what happened.

Throughout her narrative, Sarah had given several more examples of being "protected" by friends. Even before beginning the four rape narratives, Sarah described a situation with an older boy who was "trying stuff" on her in their dance class when she was 9 and he was 14. The boy would make sexual comments, "grope" her in class, and follow her to the bathroom to try to molest her. Later, she noticed that he started following her around town. She tells how there were other boys in the class who watched over her:

Yeah, he [the older boy] kept it up for 3 years, every Saturday and actually two other kids in the class caught on. They knew him and they caught on to like, you know, that he was trying stuff. . . . So they started protecting me and everything and actually one of the guys, Harry, ended up beating him up.

Sarah tells of another instance that occurred prior to the four rapes in which a boy slipped something into her drink and started "fooling around" with her after she passed out. This time, it was a girlfriend who came to her rescue:

She [her girlfriend] walked in on it, and she beat the crap out of him and kicked him out of the house and then she went back to the party.

She also discussed how others protected her even when violence was not involved. She indicated that she liked James, rather than Jack, because James watched out for her. She explained:

When I was younger I didn't smoke. James knew the smell of cigarettes bothered me and, like, all our friends smoke and, like, whenever I was around James would make all the guys put out their cigarettes. He always kept air freshener around the living room and, like, whenever I was, like, I was even at my friend's house, they were all smoking cigarettes and I was upstairs with my friend. I came downstairs, he heard me on the steps and he made all the guys put out the cigarettes and everything because he knew it bothered me.

Yet, Sarah's protectors often prove to be ineffective or disingenuous in their role. After Sam's "gallant" gesture of beating up John, for example, he then merely "threw" Sarah in the front seat of the car with John and took her home. Despite Jerry's role as Sarah's friend and protector, he also indirectly let her down. She described how she clung to him when they first got to camp, but eventually he left her to fend for herself because he wanted to spend time with other friends. It is then that she meets Alex. Jack's failings in his role as Sarah's confidant are obvious when he rapes her. Sarah's friend fends off a would-be attacker when Sarah is passed out at the party but then returns to partying, leaving Sarah as she found her. Sarah's focus on how others watched over her suggests that the quest for a protector or savior was a critical part of her rape experiences and her life. However, as occurred in the initial conditions, many of those from whom she sought protection let her down in one way or another.

Her description of the aftermath of the fourth rape differs from the other three, and from her description of other incidents involving a "protector," in one important aspect. In this narrative, it is she herself who retaliates against the rapist when she confronts Hank in the school library, protecting another young woman from being taken in, and possibly raped, by Hank. She changes roles from the protected to the protector in a public and dramatic fashion. Including a description of this incident, a different coda, in her last narrative seemed to serve to alert the audience that something has changed in the pattern of Sarah's experiences.

Sarah's Narrative as a Whole

The core narrative of each of the four rape stories is the same: Sarah is abandoned, chance events lead to her being alone with the rapist, the rape occurs despite her protests and her attempts to fight back, and she seeks a protector or confidant following each rape—only to be let down by those to whom she goes for help. The parallel form of Sarah's four rape stories thus seem to have a common purpose—all were aimed at "explaining" the reportable events. Sarah tells each story in a way that ensures that the listener is aware that it is because of misfortune that she ended up alone with the men who assaulted her and that she never desired the invasive sexual activity; rather, she was either surprised or overpowered by each rapist.

The four rape stories are tied together by the theme of abandonment and betrayal. Polkinghorne (1988) considers plot development to be a dialectic process between events and a theme that renders the events significant. Happenings are revealed as they relate to human purpose. The plot identifies the physical, cultural, and social environment that either thwarts or facilitates the human purpose and thus provides the context for action. Sarah's narrative as a whole reflects Polkinghorne's notion of dialectic process. It is the theme (abandonment and betrayal) that renders the events (the rapes) significant. If, in fact, the form of narratives reflect a "deeper" and unarticulated layer of experience (Lieblich et al., 1998), Sarah's narrative reveals that she has been forsaken by others in a fundamental way, and this is intimately tied to the violence in her life. We could not understand her experiences of rape without appreciating her experiences of being betrayed and abandoned by those close to her.

Cultural Influences on the Structure of the Narrative

Because cultural influences determine not only the content of stories but also shape the *way* we tell our stories, we need to consider the sociocultural context of Sarah's life in order to fully appreciate the meaning of her stories. Howard (1991) defined culture as "a community of individuals who see their world in a particular manner—who share particular interpretations as central to the meaning of their lives and action" (p. 190). Mair (1988) argued:

We are not only shaped by our embeddedness in the stories of our time. We are also shaped through the hidden rules of story telling that we also inherit. There are powerful structures built through our culture, in language, custom, convention, brick and stone. (p. 130)

Our culture defines what stories are fundamental in our daily lives. Children tell the dominant stories of their cultural group at young ages. Jung believed the stories we live by reside in our unconscious and are linked to the great myths that have existed throughout time (Howard, 1991).

We hear "culture tales" from a variety of sources. These tales are not only embedded in family life but pervade most of all our experience. In modern times, for example, children are continually immersed in the stories of popular culture shown on television, in movies, and in video games. The cartoons children watch "play out the external conflicts of good versus evil, issues of life and death, as well as the role of love and hate in human interactions" (Howard, 1991, p. 193).

We belong to multiple cultural subgroups (racial, socioeconomic, sexual, religious, political), all of which exert influence on us. While cultures share dominant story lines and narrative forms, stories have different meanings and implications for individuals who hear them. Multiple characters are portrayed in most stories, and individuals often identify with characters who occupy social roles similar to their own. Howard (1991) gave as an example the theatrical film *Cry Freedom,* a movie set in South Africa about a white newspaper reporter and a black anti-apartheid advocate. Howard argued that which protagonist one chooses to identify with is likely to be related to race. He explained:

The story was about friendship, oppression, and the sacrifices one makes to live out his or her values. . . . Whereas the movie clearly exalts friendship and resistance to oppression, it is instructive to inquire about what happens to people when they speak out against oppression (at least in this particular morality tale). Imagine you identified with the Black activist—he was brutally tortured and murdered by the police. The white reporter's efforts met with a rather different ending—he wrote a book about his friend which won a Pulitzer Prize and was later made into the movie *Cry Freedom.* So, after seeing that movie, will people be more likely to speak out against oppression? It depends. (p. 194)

Stories reflect the discourses of society. A discourse is "a system of statements, practices, and institutional structures that share common values" (Hare-Mustin, 1994, p. 19). Discourses sustain particular world views within a society. Freedman and Combs (1996) suggested that prevailing discourses, our cultural meta-narratives, determine what life events are storied.

These discourses both shape and are shaped by the distribution of power. Foucault (1980) argued that language is an instrument of power. The amount of power individuals have is determined by their ability to participate in the discourses that shape their society. Dominant narratives may marginalize and disempower large groups of people by excluding their voice from particular discourses. Foucault (1980) was concerned that the discourse of modern science, with its claims to truth, is dehumanizing. He sought marginalized discourses that challenged such scientific discourse and represented an "insurrection of subjugated knowledges" (Freedman & Combs, 1996, p. 237).

To consider the influence of prevailing discourses on women's stories of violence, we believe that consideration of the dominant sociocultural narrative of the patriarchy, a story that privileges men and subordinates the interests of women and children (Adams-Wescott & Isenbart, 1996), is essential. Oppression and violence against women occur in the context of this cultural narrative. Koss et al. (1994) have stressed that male violence against women is rooted in sociocultural constructions of gender and heterosexuality. They stated:

Cultural norms and expectations play critical roles promoting and shaping male violence against women, minimizing or covering up its harmful effects, and preventing the development of effective policies and programs designed to prevent such violence. Norms and expectations prescribe and proscribe the rights and responsibilities (i.e., the roles) of all persons in a particular social status or social category, including those social roles assigned by gender. It is through gender-related roles that specific cultural norms related to gender and violence are patterned, learned, and transmitted from generation to generation. Sociocultural norms and role expectations that support female subordination and perpetuate male violence are transmitted in the home, in the peer groups, at the workplace, and in the military. These norms and expectations pervade our legal system, our literary works, and our everyday discourse. (pp. 6–7)

Warshaw (1994) identified several cultural myths that influence what we believe to be true about women who are raped by men they know. These myths include: A women deserves to get raped if she is alone with a man at his home or in his car; Women who don't fight back are not really raped; If a woman lets a man buy her dinner, she owes him sex; If a women agrees to kissing or "petting," she has agreed to intercourse; When men are sexually aroused they cannot keep themselves from forcing the woman to have sex. Other cultural myths related to rape include: Women want, ask for, or deserve sexual assault; Rape only happens to certain types of women; Women often lie about rape for revenge or to protect their reputation following a regretted social encounter (Koss et al., 1994).

Several authors have argued that the discourse of social science research perpetuates violence against women by obscuring the reality of women's experiences. Jones (1994) wrote:

Domestic violence is one of those gray phrases, beloved of bureaucracy, designed to give people a way of talking about a topic without seeing what is really going on. Like repatriation or ethnic cleansing it is a euphemistic abstraction that keeps us at a dispassionate distance, far removed from the repugnant spectacle of human beings in pain. . . . We used to speak of wife beating. . . . Or we called it wife torture, the words of Frances Power Cobbe, that conjure the scenes between beatings, the sullen husband, withdrawn and sulking, or angry and intimidating, dumping dinner on the floor, throwing the cat against the wall, screaming, twisting a child's arm, needling, nagging, manipulating, criticizing the bitch, the slut, the cunt who never does anything right, who's ugly and stupid, who should keep her mouth shut, who should spread her legs now, who should be dead, who will be if she's not careful. . . . But we prefer to speak of "domestic violence." . . . [P]rofessionals in mental health and justice, equipped with professional vocabularies, took up problems of spouse abuse, conjugal violence, and marital aggression, and a great renaming took place, a renaming that veiled once again the sexism that a grass roots women's movement had worked to uncover. (p. 82)

Such arguments call for a critique of any account of intimate violence that strips the problem of its gendered context, veils institutionalized sexism, and locates the violence within individual and relationship pathology. In such accounts, the importance of social–structural factors, including gender role socialization, patriarchal systems of power, and the "trauma-generating" (Bloom, 1997) power of a society that accepts violence as a legitimate way to solve problems and create entertainment, is diminished. Many accounts of women abuse, for example, portray battered women as mentally ill and fail to demonstrate how the trauma of the assaults can *cause* post-traumatic stress.

White and Epston (1990) have argued that individuals internalize the dominant narratives of their culture, thereby forgoing their preferred narratives, because they believe that the dominant narratives reflect the truth of our identities. In Joanne's study of the meaning that battered women make of their experiences, for example, she found that the women's narratives revealed a good deal about how the selves of women are inscribed in their social reality. As stated previously, each woman told a "first time" and "worst time" story of abuse. Below are excerpts of these texts and Joanne's interpretations of what these texts reveal about the impact of culture on the lives of the women.

In the first time stories, the women spoke of the shock of being hurt by someone that they loved. These stories seemed to say, "I did not anticipate this; I did NOT ask for it in any way." Frances told of a first incident of violence:

And on the way to the place we were going to eat I asked him why he didn't get up, you know (people were waiting), and he was just cussing at me and that was the first time I remember he really gave me a good kick in the leg.

Abby provided insight into the meaning of the first time experience:

We were married for 16 years that first time when he slapped me across the face . . . but it was 3 weeks later it happened again and only a couple of weeks after that again. And that's what I said, once that barrier was broken . . . and I read that years later when there started to be more writing on that subject. I read that and I thought they're exactly right because when it happened the first time he was as shocked as I was. He couldn't believe he did that, and I really thought it would never happen again. When it happened the second time. . . . Once that barrier is broken.

The worst time stories seem to reflect the point in the relationship when the women decided that the relationship was becoming dangerous to her and that she must act. Lucia told this story of the worst time:

I can remember my worst experience was a fight that we'd had and he pushed me back and I tripped over something that was behind me. The next day, I can remember my whole armpit all the way down to my elbow was so totally bruised that I couldn't believe anyone could sustain a bruise that big on their body. That really scared me. I started to be really afraid of him.

For Frances, the worst time was a terrifying awareness of her own mortality:

[He pulled off] the road and just took his fist and just kept hitting me in the back of my head, the side of my head, and my face. I had to go to work like that. That's when I decided, "That's it!" I had it up to here and I thought I got to take care of myself. My life is precious enough. He could have hit me anywhere. The kids would have been . . . he could have been put in jail if he would have killed me or he could have put me in a nursing home or something. I could have been left a vegetable. And the kids, where were they gonna be?

Joanne concluded that the structure of the women's narratives—the universal inclusion of both first time and worst time stories—reflects the double bind women face due to the gender oppression encoded in dominant narratives of our society. In these narratives, women are expected to sustain relationships and keep them harmonious; male violence occurs only if a woman fails in these responsibilities. The women's first time stories always included a description of the shock of being physically assaulted and an emphasis that they "had done nothing to bring it on." The first time stories, therefore, served the purpose of counteracting the cultural myth that women do something, or fail to do something, that provokes the violent acts of men.

The worst time stories also reveal culturally embedded narratives. These stories were about violent episodes that were "the last straw" because they were, or had the potential to be, life threatening. These stories imply that women should take action or threaten the relationship only when the violence is "serious." Because of gender expectations that women nurture their relationships at all costs, anything they do to disrupt the relationship must be considered a "last resort."

We believe that Sarah's stories, like those of the battered women in Joanne's study, reflect the double bind women experience due to gender oppression and can only be fully understood when considered in relationship to the dominant sociocultural narrative of the patriarchy. We speculate that just as the battered women in Joanne's study needed to dispel the cultural myth that they did something to deserve the violence, Sarah had the burden of disputing the myth that women deserve to get raped if they are alone with a man in his home or in his car. She provided the level of detail she did about events leading up to the rape to emphasize that she did not simply choose to be alone with the rapist. Her narrative had to be structured so that this myth could be counteracted and her audience could appreciate that she was not to blame for the assaults.

The level of detail she provided about the rapes themselves seemed to serve to counteract the cultural myth that if a woman agrees to some sexual activity she has automatically agreed to intercourse as well. Sarah needed to convince her audience that she did not implicitly agree to the invasive sexual activity in any of the four assaults and could do nothing to stop or prevent it; she was not to be blamed for the rapes. Similar to the women interviewed by Joanne, Sarah needed to provide "evidence" that she did not ask for, deserve, or enjoy the acts committed against her.

Both sets of stories speak volumes about the nature of the shame that women experience. Bartky (1990) states:

[Women's] shame is manifest in a pervasive sense of personal inadequacy that, like the shame of embodiment, is profoundly disempowering; both reveal the "generalized condition of dishonor" which is women's lot in a sexist society. [This shame] is not so much a particular feeling or emotion . . . as a pervasive affective attunement to the social environment, that women's shame is more than merely an effect of subordination but, within the larger universe of patriarchal social relations, a profound mode of disclosure of both self and situation. (p. 85)

Estes (1992) argued that women are born with gifts of a "wildish" nature that are lost through society's attempts to civilize them into rigid roles. She stated:

A healthy woman is much like a wolf: robust, chock-full, strong life force, life-giving, territorially aware, inventive, loyal, roving. Yet, separation from the wildish nature causes a woman's personality to become meager, thin, ghostly, spectral. (p. 12)

Pipher (1994) observed a similar phenomena in her clinical practice. She wrote:

As I looked at the culture that girls enter as they come of age, I was struck by what a girl-poisoning culture it was. . . . America today limits girls' development, truncates their wholeness and leaves many of them traumatized. (p. 12)

Girls know but perhaps do not see they are losing themselves. One girl said, "Everything good in me died in junior high" (p. 20).

People who are oppressed, however, also have experiences outside of destructive dominant narratives. White and Epston (1990) called these experiences unique outcomes, which are moments when individuals are not dominated by the problems that have defined their lives. Unique outcomes are often acts of rebellion or insurrection and reveal people's competencies, autonomy, and emotional vitality—strengths that have been otherwise suppressed by oppressive forces. As mentioned above, the coda of Sarah's fourth rape story differed from the others. Rather than seeking a protector or retaliator, she confronts Hank herself in the library. This story seems to be Sarah's unique outcome.

Narrative Typologies

We next consider whether Sara's stories "fit" with any classic literary styles or existing typologies of narrative forms. The classification of narrative plots is rooted in traditional Greek drama (Gergen, 1988). The early Greeks differentiated the tragedy, the story of a fall of a noble protagonist, attributable to a "tragic flaw," and the comedy, the story of the commoner who, after a series of life challenges, experiences a happy ending.

Gergen (1988) proposed three basic plot lines according to the type of change experienced by the protagonist. In the progressive narrative, the protagonist advances steadily toward his or her goal. In the regressive narrative, the protagonist experiences deterioration or decline, moving away from his or her goal. In the stability narrative, the protagonist remains unchanged in relation to his or her goal. These basic plots are combined to form more complex narrative structures. The tragic narrative is the story of a rapid downfall of a person in a high position, that is, a progressive narrative followed by a rapid regressive narrative. The radical shift to the regressive narrative provides the dramatic power of the tragedy. The comedic narrative is the story of the trials and tribulations of the protagonist, which are unexpectedly followed by good fortune, that is, a regressive narrative followed by a progressive narrative. The dramatic power of this narrative is the critical, abrupt shift to the progressive narrative, which provides a release of emotional tension resulting from the telling of the progressive decline. A progressive narrative followed by a stability narrative is considered a "happily ever after" narrative, the most soothing type of story line. A romantic saga is a series of progressive–regressive phases. Gergen suggested that such schemas may be applied to the narratives people tell about their lives, arguing that "by asking questions about these various aspects of the narrative, the researcher may develop several ways to extend psychological inquiry" (p. 102).

Narrative Typologies of Stories of Suffering

While we did not uncover any narrative typologies for stories related to violence, we found two such typologies for illness stories, which, as stated earlier, we have come to believe are similar in nature to trauma stories. Frank (1995) described three types of illness narratives, each reflecting a different cultural or personal preference.

Frank's Types of Illness Narratives

Restitution Narrative   The restitution plot reflects society's assumption that health is normal and thus ought to be restored. Because illness is viewed as transitory, mortality is not of concern. The plot of the restitution narrative, the "good as new" scenario, is as follows: "Yesterday I was healthy, today I'm sick, but tomorrow I will be healthy again" (Frank, 1995, p. 72). This narrative is exemplified by the television commercial for nonprescription drugs. The typical plot depicts first an episode of misery and social default, followed by consumption of the "remedy," ending with the restoration of physical comfort and the resumption of expected duties.

In the restitution narrative, the illness interruption is finite and remediable; one's future is not threatened. The present illness is an aberration in an otherwise normal passage of time. Responsibility involves taking medicine and getting well. Restitution does not depend on the struggles of the self but rather on the advances of modern medicine. These narratives are about the heroism of applied science.

Frank (1995) argued that restitution stories represent the culturally preferred narrative and may crowd out other narratives. If these narratives do not "work"—if health is not restored—those who are dying or who are chronically ill may not have alternative narratives to fall back on. Because confrontation with mortality cannot be a part of the restitution story, the seriously ill are left with a plot with no meaningful ending.

The Chaos Narrative   Frank (1995) envisioned the chaos plot as the opposite of the restitution plot; it is about a life that will never get better. The chaos story depicts life experiences that are without coherent sequence or sense of causality. "Chaos stories are sucked into the undertow of illness and the disasters that attend to it" (p. 115). Chaos stories are of immediate frustrations, insults, and agonies. The plot takes the form of "and then, and then, and then." Frank stated:

In these stories the modernist bulwark of remedy, progress, and professionalism cracks to reveal vulnerability, futility, and impotence. If the restitution narrative promises possibilities of outdistancing or outwitting suffering, the chaos narrative tells how easily any of us could be sucked under. (p. 97)

The chaos narrative is the most embodied form of the story—the hole in the telling. Because lived chaos makes reflection impossible, these stories are in a sense anti-narratives but can be pieced together from fragments of the ill person's communications.

Frank (1995) stressed, however, that we need to listen to and honor these stories. In our culture, we tend to focus on the resiliency of the human spirit, leaving no room for the chaos narrative. Because the chaos story is not the culturally preferred narrative, it causes anxiety for the listener. Listeners tend to believe that if they fall into a chaos story, they would never find a way out. Our reluctance to hear chaos stories limits the ability of the teller to find recognition or support for pain and suffering.

The Quest Narrative   Quest narratives are stories about meeting illness head on (Frank, 1995). The illness becomes a journey that takes the form of a quest. Ill persons retain their own voices and become the heroes of their own stories. Something is always gained from the quest.

Joseph Campbell (1972) described the narrative structure of the quest story, which occurs in three stages. The first stage is the departure, which begins with a "call." In illness narratives, the call is often a physical symptom—be it a pain, a lump, or a cough. Because the ill person is aware of the suffering ahead, the call is often "refused"—the symptom is denied or ignored. When the call can no longer be refused, the "first threshold" is crossed and the ill person, who now becomes the hero, enters the stage of initiation. The threshold may involve hospitalization or surgery resulting in a diagnosis. The initiation is called the "road of trials," as it involves physical, emotional, and spiritual suffering. The road may involve other stages, such as temptation or atonement. Through the process of the journey, the hero experiences a transformation. She or he gains something from the experience, often a profound insight, that must then be passed onto others. The final stage, the end, occurs when the illness is gone, but the hero is forever changed. The return necessitates the hero being a witness to the integrity of suffering.

Frank (1995) identified three types of quest stories: the memoir, manifesto, and automythology. The memoir is an illness story told within the context of other events in the storyteller's life; memoirs represent an interrupted autobiography. Trials are told stoically with no dramatic insight; rather, the plot reflects the incorporation of illness into the person's life story. Memoirs are often told by the famous; the subtext of the story is the split between the glamour of the public persona and the reality of the illness.

The manifesto, on the other hand, highlights prophetic insights that demand social action. Because the truth about illness is suppressed by society, those who are ill are obliged to tell their stories. One's "former health" is considered an illusion, and therefore restoration is not valued. Suffering is used to enlighten others and provoke them to action. Illness is a social issue not a personal affliction. The manifesto "witnesses how society has added to the physical problems that disease entails, and it calls for change based on solidarity of the afflicted" (Frank, 1995, p. 122). Frank's description of the manifesto resembles Tierney's (2000) discussion of a testimony. Tierney stated that a testimony is "developed by the one who testifies in the hope that his or her life story will move the reader to action in concert with the group with which the testifier identifies" (p. 540). The purpose of the testimony is social change; there is a moral imperative for the author, who typically is a silenced, marginalized, or oppressed member of society, to tell the story. The author does not rise above the struggle, but rather remains connected to those who also suffer.

The third type of the quest narrative is the automythology; these are stories of self-reinvention. The hero not only survives but is reborn; he or she defines a new existence. Unlike the manifesto, the focus of these narratives is on individual change, not political reform.

Crossley's Types of Illness Narratives

Crossley (1999) proposed that HIV positive individuals use three dominant cultural narratives to tell their stories of illness: the "normalising" story, the "conversion/growth" story, and the "loss" story. Each of these types of narratives include characteristic themes, images, and metaphors that construct the experience of living with HIV in significantly different ways, each with important implications for adaptation.

The Normalising Story   In the normalising story, storytellers portray themselves as minimally affected by their illness. They speak of keeping busy, carrying on, and doing normal things. Despite their claim that the impact of their illness has been minimal, they often credit their advocacy activities for their well-being.

The Conversion/Growth Narrative   In the conversion/growth narrative, similar to Frank's (1995) automythology, ill persons obtain insight and experience a transformation as a result of their illnesses. They often decide to focus on psychological or emotional needs that were neglected in favor of physical, social, or material needs prior to their diagnosis.

These individuals may speak of giving up their old self-defeating habits and replacing them with more life-affirming activities.

The Loss Story   The third cultural narrative is the loss story. Individuals tell stories of only what they have lost by their illness; they are stories of lives destroyed. These are the stories that are tied to depression and suicidal thoughts.

Sarah's Narrative: Of What Narrative Type?

Sarah's narrative shares some features of the types of illness and suffering narratives described above but differs in some fundamental ways. Her narrative least resembles the restitution narrative as described by Frank (1995). A restitution narrative implies that illness is transitory, finite, and remediable, and health can be restored. In Sarah's narrative, violence is neither transitory, finite, or remediable. A restitution narrative may be told by a woman who has a happy and protected childhood, experiences an unexpected episode of violence, gets help from the institutions charged with aiding her and from those who love her, and returns once again to a carefree, secure life. In our experience, such narratives are rare. In much of our research, women stress that the effects of violence last a lifetime. In fact, women who suffer from violence and abuse face an ongoing paradox; the violence that prompts their search for a safer life also teaches them that their social world can be dangerous (Draucker & Stern, 2000). Life never really goes back to "the way it was."

Sarah's story is initially reminiscent of Frank's (1995) chaos narrative as it focused primarily on insults, frustrations, and agonies. Sarah says, "Since I've been little, I've always [been having] people try stuff on me." Two features of the chaos narrative are the syntactic structure of: "and then, and then, and then" (one trial and tribulation after another) and over-determination—a sense that "what can be told . . . only begins to suggest all this is wrong" (p. 99). Both of these features are evident in Sarah's plot as she relates instance after instance of maltreatment, violence, and abuse and states that she could never describe all the times she was victimized by men in one interview.

Sarah rarely considers seeking help from institutions, perhaps because professionals are prone to value those who tell a restitution narrative. Frank (1995) argued that medical professionals have difficulty witnessing the chaos narrative. He stated, "The anxiety that the chaos story provokes in others leads to the standard clinical dismissal of chaos stories as documenting 'depression.' When chaos is thus redefined as a treatable condition, the restitution narrative is restored" (p. 110). However, the person's experience is denied and the chaos may be compounded.

While Sarah's story has elements of a chaos narrative, it is not a "pure" chaos narrative as described by Frank (1995). Frank argued that individuals who are living a chaos story cannot put it into words—lived chaos has only immediacy. "The chaos that can be told in story is already taking place at a distance and is being reflected retrospectively" (p. 98). Of course, the context of Sarah's telling, the research interview, demanded reflection and resulted in a narrative with a coherent sequence that Frank suggested is typically missing in the chaos narrative. When Sarah asks where she should begin, Claire said, "Why don't you start at the beginning. . . ." Yet, even beyond context demands, Sarah's narrative transcends the chaos narrative. A chaos story lacks a sense of purpose and, as we've noted above, Sarah's narrative seems full of purpose. She tells us how bad her life has been but provides the coherence and detail needed to place her experience in its social context and forestall any suggestion that she brought on the violence.

As mentioned earlier, Roberts (1999) argued that there is a reciprocal relationship between the stories we tell and those told to us through our childhood. The "culture tale" that Sarah's narratives initially seemed to emulate is the classic Western fairy tale in which a vulnerable woman is rescued by a hero who either saves her from evil and harm or defends her honor. As mentioned above, Sarah's stories reflect an ongoing quest for such a hero. This tale is rooted in the dominant cultural meta-narrative of the patriarchy where it is the duty of the strong male to rescue the vulnerable female; that is, the white knight champions the damsel in distress. Yet, in reality, Sarah never gets the fairy tale ending of the selfless and brave savior. Her champions either let her down or further victimize her.

Sarah's description of her confrontation with Hank in the school library represented a change in her "plot." In this instance, she herself took action against the rapist and in the process protected another young woman. She takes on the role of hero and protector:

One day I ran into him [Hank] at the college library. And there was this little girl that I always saw around campus. Sweetest little thing on the face of the earth, but shy. Horribly, horribly shy. I saw him and he went over and he sat down and introduced himself to her, starting talking to her. It's not my business, really. But, um, he went over and he sat down and introduced himself to this girl and all of a sudden it hit me, I was just like, "Oh no, no, no, no, no, no." And I saw him sit down and it just triggered me. I'm like, "Oh my gosh. She doesn't have any friends." And I was just like, you know, she would be the easiest person, you know, to get. He was talking to her and I walked over to the table and I just leaned across the table and I said to her, "Get the hell away from him. He's a rapist." And she got up and she bolted. And then I said it out loud and like everybody got quiet. And he just got up and he said something like, "Fuck you" or something like that and he just walked away.

As mentioned previously, this action seems to be a "unique outcome" as described by White and Epston (1990) insofar as Sarah finds her voice and clearly takes a stand against "oppression." It is tempting to portray Sarah's narrative as a comedic narrative as defined by Gergen (1988)— a story in which the trials and tribulations of the protagonist are followed by good fortune. Even after this episode with Hank, however, Sarah continues to be maltreated by men. While she described no further sexual assaults, at the time of the interview she continued to experience some emotional and physical abuse in her current relationships.

Her narrative does suggest, however, that things did begin to change for her around this time. She had confided in and found considerable support from other women who had experienced abuse and maltreatment. She had begun to establish a relationship with her mother, who had become sober through participation in Alcoholics Anonymous. In fact, for the first time, Sarah was able to tell her mother that she had been raped. Sarah also found a therapist who was helpful to her.

Her narrative began to resemble, in some regards, a quest narrative, especially the automythology as described by Frank (1995). Sarah reveals that because of her personal experiences with violence and abuse, she has gained insight that she passes on to others. At several points late in her interview she expressed concern about other women who had never experienced abuse because these women were not aware of real dangers lurking in the world. She described one incident in which she and a friend went to a bar and the friend decided to leave with a man:

And she [her friend] literally, she's never had a bad experience before in her life. When I met her—she just lost her virginity a couple months prior—and like never had any guys try to go further with her. Like she's been real lucky.

She totally thinks she's untouchable and I ended up having to go with her, and he's a harmless guy. He was harmless. But it was just . . . like I tried to explain to her. I told her "Just don't take off with people like that. Don't meet people at a bar and go home with them that night. You don't know them. You don't know what you're going to walk in on or like. . . ." So you know when I meet girls I will talk with them. And like I'll inform people, you know.

Sarah explains that she takes on this role with younger women because of what she has learned in her own personal experience. She stated, "You learn off what you've gone through and what could happen to you. And you, like, learn the do's and the don'ts and where you can go and how to act and so on. But we also learn what kind of guys we want in our lives." As Estes (1992) claimed:

All creatures must learn that there exist predators. Without this knowing, a woman will be unable to negotiate safely within her own forest without being devoured. To understand the predator is to become a mature animal who is not vulnerable out of naivete . . . (p. 46)

Sarah never suggests, however, that she has experienced a profound change because of her experience with violence, as would be the case in a "pure" quest narrative, but rather that throughout her life she has learned many "hard" lessons she now chooses to pass on. Kleinman (1988) referred to the work of William James on the two kinds of practical personal perspectives on experience. Kleinman explained:

The once born James took to be native optimists who tended to see everyday life and religion on the surface: hopeful, positive, well-ordered, progressive. The twice born, in contrast, were most pessimistic. They tended to focus on the darker underside of experience. The twice born were absorbed by questions of social injustice and personal pain. (p. 54)

Kleinman argued that chronic illness converts the once born into the twice born. We argue the same is true for violence. Violence teaches that there is undesired and undeserved suffering. Women who experience violence apprehend the dark side of human relationships.

Sarah's narrative thus has elements of both a chaos and a quest narrative but is perhaps best described as a narrative of the twice born. She knows she must convince us that she did not ask to be raped, was not to blame, and did not consent to the invasive sexual activities. She attempted to fit her story into the culture tale of the endangered woman and the savior, but her experiences revealed the inadequacy of this narrative. Instead, as is typical in the narratives of the twice born, she describes an "insight [that is the result] of an often grim, though occasionally luminous, lived wisdom of the body in pain and the mind troubled" (Kleinman, 1988, p. 22).

Summary

Because the essence of human thought is revealed in the stories we tell (Howard, 1991), appreciating narrative knowledge is crucial to understanding the human experience. The narrative analysis of Sarah's interview does support Lieblich and colleagues' (1998) suggestion that the formal aspects of narrative structure shed much light on the storyteller's identity and perceptions and reveal a great deal about how culture influences the act of storytelling itself. The manner in which Sarah structured the four rape narratives, and how she embedded those narratives within her life story, says much about her inner world and her social reality. For Sarah, violence is intimately tied to abandonment and betrayal. Although she seeks the savior promised to her in the fairy tales told to little girls in this culture and in the romance novels sold to adult women, these characters never materialize.

Sarah is left with the burden of explaining why she was abused and maltreated most of her life. She must explain how she ended up alone with the rapists in order to convince us she did not ask to be raped, and she must emphasize how she fought back to convince us that she did not enjoy the sexual aggression. She cannot simply say that she lives in a violent and oppressive society, in a social world in which children are abandoned and females of all ages are violated and abused; that is not the culturally preferred narrative. In fact, we feared that Sarah's story may be interpreted by some as the story of a woman "prone" to violence, or even worse, "asking for it," because she was raped four times. However, this conclusion is possible only if the historical and social contexts of her narrative and Sarah's own words were ignored. She wanders the streets alone as a young child and is periodically taken in by strangers, but her plight never comes to the attention of those charged with protecting children, and her parents are never held accountable for their neglect. John, Alex, Jack, and Hank have sex with her without her permission and against her desire. She never entertains the possibility of reporting the attacks; these are "nice" guys, and she knows it is "my word against theirs."

Sarah's story is not one of restitution (a happy ending provided to her by society's institutions), nor one of only chaos (a woman "destined" to violence "again" and "again"), nor one of only quest (a romantic journey resulting in transforming enlightenment). Sarah's story was one of suffering and survival and the sad wisdom she acquired about human nature and the world in which she lives. Sarah's story is a narrative of the twice born; her story provokes critique of the dark side of a social world in which violence and oppression goes unchecked, a dark side of which she has knowledge because of her lived experience.

While existing typologies of illness narratives provided a useful starting point for us, Sarah's story suggests that women's narratives of violence may differ from other tales of suffering. Violence against women results from acts of agency, rather than facticity, and occurs within a context of gender oppression. For this project, we focused on one woman's narrative. Examining the narratives of many women who have experienced violence and oppression could yield a typology that reflects a diversity of perspectives and cultural influences.

Stories are interpretations of experience, not descriptions alone, and people choose the form of the story based on what they need to do, to achieve, as well as what they have lived, personally and culturally. Sarah needed to contradict a dominant cultural narrative, with all the myths that accompany it, to reveal her experiences and depict her lifeworld. Sarah was summoned to tell her story, not by the researcher, but by her uninterpreted experiences—her "wild logos." Had we only dissected her narrative or abstracted her experiences, we might have not heard the story she chose to tell or appreciated the narrative strategies she used to get her point across.

Implications for Healthcare Professionals

Stories are important. They keep us alive. In the ships, in the camps, in the quarters, fields, prisons, on the road, on the run, underground, under siege, in the throes, on the verge—the storyteller snatches us back from the edge to hear the next chapter. In which we are the subjects. We, the hero of the tales. Our lives preserved. How it was; how it be. Passing it along in the relay. That is what I work to do: to produce stories that save our lives. (Bambara, 1984, p. 41)

Stories *are* important. They *can* be what keeps us alive, after being twice born through suffering. Perhaps the most obvious implication of Sarah's stories is the call for healthcare providers to listen *differently* to the stories of those who have experienced violence, abuse, or oppression. Sarah had a story to tell that had been silenced by therapists charged with helping her—those "stern older women" who looked as if they "were going to choke" when she tried to tell them how she was suffering. Much has been written about the silencing of those who have experienced violence or trauma. Roberts (1999) argued:

For some, the issue is not that a story is fractured, mysterious or lost but that it cannot be spoken. The individual believes his experiences to be so unacceptable to others, or risk such negative reactions, that they are held with fear and shame, concealed, or hidden. (p. 19)

As Frank (1995) pointed out, healthcare providers may be especially reluctant to hear stories that are inconsistent with culturally preferred narratives. He argued that the restitution narrative is the preferred illness story. Stories of repeated abuse and ongoing suffering, that is, stories of chaos, are not of this genre and may be excluded from healthcare discourse. Yet, the telling of stories of trauma has been shown to be associated with improved health. Pennebaker and colleagues, for example, have shown that writing about personally traumatic events in a laboratory setting is associated with varied health benefits, evidenced by lowered healthcare utilization, fewer absentee days, and improved liver enzyme function (Pennebaker, 1993; Pennebaker & Beall, 1986; Pennebaker, Colder, & Sharp, 1990; Pennebaker, Kiecolt-Glaser, & Glaser, 1988).

Mental health clinicians have long maintained that individuals who have experienced traumatic events need to tell their stories as part of their healing. Many therapeutic modalities consider catharsis, the emotional release that accompanies the telling of life's painful experiences, to be a critical element of therapeutic change (Prochaska & Norcross, 1994). Contemporary models of trauma treatment are based on the telling and retelling of the traumatic experiences, not merely for emotional release but to foster integration of dissociated memories that return as intrusive experiences or troubling images. Courtois (1999) stated: "The primary goal of trauma resolution and integration is for the patient to gradually face and make sense of the abuse/trauma and to experience associated emotions at a pace that is safe, manageable, and not over-whelming" (p. 203). Brown, Scheflin, and Hammond (1998) proposed that describing threatening events from the past "is about mastery over what has been unclear or avoided in memory, making meaning out of one's personal history, and achieving integration" (p. 481).

Clearly, stories of trauma need to be told, but little has been written about how healthcare providers may best listen and respond. In Claire's research project on women's responses to sexual violence by male inti-mates, all the women thought that telling others about the violence was crucial to their recovery, but different women believed that different kinds of "talk" were helpful (Draucker & Stern, 2000). Women who had experienced isolated incidents of violence by a man whom they did not know well, such as a new boyfriend, coworker, or acquaintance, wanted "reassuring talk" from others; they wanted validation that what hap-pened to them was rape and reassurance that the rape was not their fault. This also appeared to be true for the women that Joanne spoke to in her study. They did not want advice about what to do, such as whether or not to report the assault to the authorities.

Women who were assaulted by a man who was close to them, such as a husband or long-time partner, over a period of time, wanted "moti-vating talk" from others; they wanted to be told that they did not deserve the abuse and were worthy of being treated well. They wanted others to "plant the seeds of change" without insisting they leave the relationship (Draucker & Stern, 2000).

Women who experienced much abuse and violence throughout their lives starting in childhood wanted "restoring talk" from others; they needed talk that was not just reassuring or motivating but talk that could repair damage done to their sense of self by years of abuse. These women recognized that restoring talk had to "go back," "dig deep," or "get to the core of the problem" (Draucker & Stern, 2000). Thus, while telling about trauma can be healing, not all responses by others may be equally helpful. When responding to stories of violence, healthcare professionals may need to consider the historical and situational context of the abuse.

Healthcare providers also need a better understanding of stories that individuals tell themselves. As Terry Waite argued, in desperate life-threatening circumstances, telling stories to oneself may be life sus-taining. Harvey and colleagues (Orbuch, Harvey, Davis, & Merbach,

1994; Weber & Harvey, 1994) argued that the private experience of formulating an account of loss and trauma and the public experience of disclosing it to others both contribute to recovery from loss. Much has been written about the healing effects of disclosing traumatic stories to others, but we know little about the "subjective experience of chronicling, confirming, and translating strong emotions and memories into symbolic images" (Bochner, Ellis, & Tillman-Healy, 2000, p. 24).

The notion that life events are told to others, and to oneself, in narrative form has important implications for health professionals. Our findings suggest that healthcare providers should consider what the narrative structure of the story might reveal about the storyteller's experience and that this may require providers to rethink their previously held assumptions about how they listen to stories and, even more profoundly, the function of this listening in the treatment of the teller. Our interpretation of the structure of Sarah's narrative, for example, included our lament that Sarah needed to justify and explain the sexual assaults she experienced because her story did not reflect the canonical story of her culture, that is, the story of the rescued and protected princess. Bochner and colleagues (2000) argued that individuals "feel a strong need to explain, justify, excuse, or legitimize" (p. 20) their own choices and actions when their stories deviate from the cultural norm.

We recommend that healthcare providers respond to stories in a way that somehow lifts the burden of reconciling one's life experiences with the preferred culture tale. The question is: How can individuals be freed from the walls of canonical stories and be encouraged to become authors, rather than carriers, of their own stories (Bochner et al., 2000)? To begin to answer this question, providers may need to wrangle with postmodern questions about the nature of "truth." A detailed discussion of this topic is beyond the scope of this chapter. However, we refer here to the beliefs and related practices of providers who think that it is important for them and for the storyteller to get the story "straight," to find the "Truth" (with a capital "T"), or to uncover the "reality" of the situation. While this may be important in the prosecution of crimes related to assaults women have endured, it can be stifling when they try to tell their stories. As mentioned earlier, Claire noted that, with regard to her research practices, getting information is not the same as creating a space for a story to be told and to be heard. This is equally true in clinical practice.

Narrative therapy is one treatment approach that seeks to make visible the ways in which people's stories are shaped by the social and historical context of their lives, making way for the construction of life stories that are meaningful and fulfilling. Although a description of the specific techniques of this approach are beyond the scope of this discussion and have been reviewed elsewhere (White, 1989, 1995; White & Epston, 1990), we do believe that the assumptions of narrative therapy suggest new ways to listen to stories that are laden with suffering and crowded with justification. The basic premise of narrative therapy is that individuals often internalize a dominant, yet oppressive, cultural narrative that prevents them from living out their preferred life story, and the goal is to free them from the constraints of the destructive narrative in order to open up the possibilities for the creation of a new life story. As described earlier, individuals whose lives are dominated by suffering and saturated with abuse often describe events representing "unique outcomes," experiences inconsistent with the dominant narrative of oppression (Freedman & Combs, 1996). These events, such as Sarah's confrontation of Hank in the library, deviate from the plot of problem-saturated narratives and reflect "little pockets of non-cooperation, moments of personal courage and autonomy, self-respect and emotional vitality beneath the iron grid of lived misery and assigned pathology" (Wylie, 1994, p. 43). If healthcare providers can bring forth such often-hidden stories, a space for a new narrative may be opened. Therapeutic approaches that encourage disempowered or marginalized individuals to question the dominant narrative and support their personal insurrection against oppression offer healthcare providers different ways of listening to, and calling forth, stories.

Another narrative approach that we are drawn to places the healthcare professional in the role of the storyteller. Gersie (1997) discussed how traditional tales may be told by the therapist to connect old stories with life experiences. She argued that individuals "demand that stories be a good yarn, something to while away the time or to offer inspiration, whilst possibly quietly hoping that it might address the central, underlying story of their own life, to grant it at least a semblance of coherency and to illuminate its purpose" (p. 14). Estes (1992) described how multicultural, women-centered myths and folk tales can be told to help women reconnect with their feminine, instinctual archetype. She stated:

Although some use stories as entertainment alone, tales are, in their oldest sense, a healing art. Some are called to this healing art, and the best, to my lights, are those who have lain with the story and found all its matching parts inside themselves and at depth. (p. 463)

Estes tells the Russian folk tale of Vasalisa. Vasalisa is given a doll by her dying mother. Vasalisa is to feed and nourish the doll; the doll will in return provide advice and guidance to Vasalisa. Vasalisa's father re-marries, and, like the Western tale of Cinderella, Vasalisa's selfish step-mother and stepsisters treat her cruelly, making her life one of drudgery. Vasalisa is sent to Baba Yaga, a murderous Hag, under the pretense of getting fire to warm the family's home and cook their food; the step-mother and sisters actually expect that Baba Yaga will kill and eat Vasa-lisa. Baba Yaga imposes on Vasalisa a number of dangerous tasks that she must accomplish in return for her life and the fire. Vasalisa meets her trials and is granted the fire; the fire ultimately consumes the step-mother and sisters, ending Vasalisa's torment. Estes suggests that Vasa-lisa is saved, not by Prince Charming, but by the strength and inde-pendence she secures from the women in her life: her mother, who bequeaths her the doll that serves as her guiding intuition; the step-mother, who forces her out of the house, thereby ending her victimiza-tion; and Baba Yaga, from whom she learns of her own awesome power. Stories such as this, therefore, may provide alternatives to tales that idealize men as saviors and protectors and facilitate women in creating their own women-centered life tales.

A vital way of helping survivors hear the stories of others is to con-nect them to resources where the ongoing creative and developmental activity of conversation and storytelling takes place. For people who have been raped and battered, programs of services exist throughout the United States that offer support groups where stories of suffering and survival are told and heard. Healthcare providers can find these resources by calling their local domestic violence and sexual assault programs or by contacting the National Domestic Violence Hotline at: 1-800-799-SAFE [7233] or on the web at: www.ndvh.org, or the Na-tional Sexual Violence Resource Center at: 877-739-3895 or on the web at: www.nsvrc.org.

Healthcare professionals will receive stories of suffering; it is funda-mental to the work that we do. We encourage healthcare professionals to remain open to the healing potential of stories and become familiar with what narratives may reveal about the life experiences of those for whom they provide care. Through our research and clinical practice we have been reminded of how we must create a particular kind of space, both physically and interpersonally, for stories to be told and heard. We believe that to create this space we must confront our deeply ingrained habits and practices of information-gathering, developing instead new ways of listening and responding to the stories of the twice born. In this way, healthcare providers can join with survivors of abuse and violence as they produce new life narratives—stories that will preserve all of our lives.

References

Adams-Wescott, J., & Isenbart, D. (1996). Creating preferred relationships: The politics of recovery from child sexual abuse. *Journal of Systemic Therapies, 15*(1), 13–30.

Antaki, C. (1994). *Explaining and arguing: The social organization of accounts.* Thousand Oaks, CA: Sage.

Bambara, T. C. (1984). Salvation is the issue. In M. Evans (Ed.), *Black women writers: 1950–1980* (p. 41). New York: Anchor Doubleday Books.

Bartky, S. (1990). *Femininity and domination: Studies in the phenomenology of oppression.* New York: Routledge.

Bell, S. E. (1988). Becoming a political woman: The reconstruction and interpretation of experience through stories. In A. D. Todd & S. Fisher (Eds.), *Gender and discourse: The power of talk* (pp. 97–123). Norwood, NJ: Ablex.

Bloom, S. (1997). *Creating sanctuary: Toward an evolution of sane societies.* New York: Routledge.

Bochner, A. P., Ellis, C., & Tillman-Healey, L. M. (2000). Relationships as stories: Accounts, stories lives, evocative narratives. In K. Dindia & S. Duck (Eds.), *Communication and personal relationships* (pp. 13–29). New York: John Wiley & Sons.

Brown, D., Scheflin, A. W., & Hammond, D. C. (1998). *Memory, trauma treatment, and the law: An essential reference on memory for clinicians, researchers, attorneys, and judges.* New York: Norton.

Bruner, J. (1990). *Acts of meaning.* Cambridge, MA: Harvard University Press.

Campbell, J. (1972). *The hero with a thousand faces.* Princeton, NJ: Princeton University Press.

Chase, S. E. (1995). Taking narrative seriously: Consequences for method and theory in interview studies. In R. Josselson & A. Lieblich (Eds.), *Interpreting experience: The narrative study of lives* (pp. 1–26). Thousand Oaks, CA: Sage.

Chatwin, B. (1988). *The songlines.* London: Picador.

Coles, R. (1989). *The call of stories.* Boston: Houghton Mifflin.

Courtois, C. A. (1999). *Recollections of sexual abuse: Treatment principles and guidelines.* New York: Norton.

Crossley, M. L. (1999). Stories of illness and trauma survival: Liberation or repression. *Social Science & Medicine, 48,* 1685–1695.

Draucker, C. B. (1992). The healing process of adult survivors of incest: Constructing a personal residence. *Image: The Journal of Nursing Scholarship, 24*(1), 4–8.

Draucker, C. B. (1999). Knowing what to do: Coping with sexual violence by male intimates. *Qualitative Health Research, 9*(5), 473–484.

Draucker, C. B., & Madsen, C. (1999). Women dwelling with violence. *Image: Journal of Nursing Scholarship, 31*(9), 327–332.

Draucker, C. B., & Stern, P. N. (2000). Women's responses to sexual violence by male intimates. *Western Journal of Nursing Research, 22*(4), 385–406.

Estes, C. P. (1992). *Women who run with wolves.* New York: Ballantine Books.

Foucault, M. (1980). *Power/knowledge: Selected interviews and other writings, 1972–1977.* New York: Pantheon Books.

Frank, A. (1995). *The wounded storyteller.* Chicago: The University of Chicago Press.

Freedman, J., & Combs, G. (1996). *Narrative therapy: The shared construction of preferred realities.* New York: Norton.

Gergen, K. J., & Gergen, M. M. (1986). Narrative form and the construction of psychological science. In T. R. Sarbin (Ed.), *Narrative psychology: The storied nature of human conduct* (pp. 22–44). New York: Praeger.

Gergen, M. M. (1988). Narrative structures in social explanation. In C. Antaki (Ed.), *Analysing everyday explanation: A casebook of methods* (pp. 94–112). Newbury Park, CA: Sage.

Gersie, A. (1997). *Reflections on therapeutic storytelling: The use of stories in groups.* Bristol, PA: Jessica Kingsley.

Hare-Mustin, R. (1994). A feminist approach to family therapy. *Family Process, 17,* 181–194.

Harvey, J. H., Orbuch, T. L., Chwalisz, K. D., & Garwood, G. (1991). Coping with sexual assault: The roles of account-making and confiding. *Journal of Traumatic Stress, 4,* 515–531.

Hessmiller, J. M. (1998). For our own good: The meaning of batterer intervention programs for women who have been abused—a Heideggerian hermeneutic inquiry. Ann Arbor, MI: University Microfilms No. 9835429.

Howard, G. S. (1991). Culture tales: A narrative approach to thinking, cross-cultural psychology, and psychotherapy. *American Psychologist, 46,* 187–197.

Jones, A. (1994). *Next time she'll be dead.* Boston: Beacon Press.

Kermode, F. (1967). *The sense of an ending: Studies in the theory of fiction.* New York: Oxford University Press.

Kleinman, A. (1988). *The illness narratives: Suffering, healing, and the human condition.* New York: Basic Books.

Koss, M. P., Goodman, L. A., Browne, A., Fitzgerald, L. F., Keita, G. P., & Russo, N. F. (1994). *Male violence against women at home, at work, and in the community.* Washington, DC: American Psychological Association.

Labov, W. (1982). Speech actions and reactions in personal narratives. In D. Tanner (Ed.), *Analyzing discourse: Text and talk* (pp. 219–247). Washington, DC: Georgetown University Press.

Lieblich, A., Tuval-Mashiach, R., & Zilber, T. (1998). *Narrative research: Reading, analysis, and interpretation.* Thousand Oaks, CA: Sage.

Mair, M. (1988). Psychology as storytelling. *International Journal of Personal Construct Psychology, 1,* 125–137.

Merleau-Ponty, M. (1962). *Phenomenology of perception* (C. Smith, Trans.). New York: Humanities Press. (Original work published 1945)

Mishler, E. G. (1986). The analysis of interview-narratives. In T. R. Sarbin (Ed.), *Narrative psychology: The storied nature of human conduct* (pp. 233–255). New York: Praeger.

Orbuch, T. L., Harvey, J. H., Davis, S. H., & Merbach, N. J. (1994). Account-making and confiding as acts of meaning in response to sexual assault. *Journal of Family Violence, 9*(3), 249-264.

Pennebaker, J. W. (1993). Putting stress into words: Health, linguistic, and therapeutic implications. *Behavioral Research and Therapy, 31*, 539–548.

Pennebaker, J. W., & Beall, S. K. (1986). Confronting a traumatic event: Toward an understanding of inhibition and disease. *Journal of Abnormal Psychology, 95*, 274–281.

Pennebaker, J. W., Colder, M., & Sharp, L. K. (1990). Accelerating the coping process. *Journal of Personality and Social Psychology, 58*, 528–537.

Pennebaker, J. W., Kiecolt-Glaser, J. & Glaser, R. (1988). Disclosure of traumas and immune function: Health implications for psychotherapy. *Journal of Consulting and Clinical Psychology, 56*, 239–245.

Pipher, M. (1994). *Reviving Ophelia*. New York: Ballantine Books.

Polkinghorne, D. E. (1988). *Narrative knowing and the human sciences*. Albany: State University of New York Press.

Prochaska, J. O., & Norcross, J. C. (1994). *Systems of psychotherapy: A transtheoretical approach*. Pacific Grove, CA: Pacific Grove.

Roberts, G. (1999). Introduction: A story of stories. In G. Roberts & J. Holmes (Eds.), *Healing stories: Narrative in psychiatry and psychotherapy* (pp. 3–26). New York: Oxford University Press.

Taylor, D. (1996). *The healing power of stories*. New York: Doubleday.

Tierney, W. G. (2000). Undaunted courage: Life history and the postmodern challenge. In N. K. Denzin & Y. S. Lincoln (Eds.), *Handbook of qualitative research* (pp. 537–555). Thousand Oaks, CA: Sage.

Warshaw, R. (1994). *I never called it rape*. New York: HarperPerennial.

Weber, A. L, & Harvey, J. H. (1994). Accounts in coping with relationship loss. In A. L. Weber & J. H. Harvey (Eds.), *Perspectives on close relationships* (pp. 285–306). Needham Heights, MA: Allyn & Bacon.

White, M. (1989). *Selected papers*. Adelaide, Australia: Dulwich Center Publications.

White, M. (1995). *Reauthoring lives: Interviews and essays*. Adelaide, Australia: Dulwich Center Publications.

White, M., & Epston, D. (1990). *Narrative means to a therapeutic end*. New York: Norton.

Wylie, M. (1994). Panning for gold. *The Family Therapy Networker, 18*(6), 40–48.

Contributors
Index

Contributors

Nancy L. Diekelmann is Helen Denne Schulte Professor at the University of Wisconsin–Madison School of Nursing, a fellow in the American Academy of Nursing, past president of the Society for Research in Nursing Education, and chair of the University of Wisconsin–Madison Teaching Academy. A noted authority for her work in nursing education and primary healthcare, Dr. Diekelmann has received two Book of the Year awards from the *American Journal of Nursing* for her textbooks *Primary Health Care of the Well Adult* and *Transforming RN Education: Dialogue and Debate* (co-authored with Marsha L. Rather). Her current research uses interpretive phenomenology to explicate the narratives of teachers, students, and clinicians in nursing education. Dr. Diekelmann has described an alternative approach for nursing education—narrative pedagogy. She is co-author with J. Diekelmann of a forthcoming book, *Schooling Learning Teaching: Toward a Narrative Pedagogy.*

Claire Burke Draucker is professor and the director of the graduate program in psychiatric–mental health nursing at Kent State University College of Nursing. She is a licensed psychologist in the State of Ohio and a Certified Clinical Specialist in Psychiatric Mental Health Nursing. Dr. Draucker has conducted studies on early family experiences and later victimization in the lives of women, the healing processes of women and men who were sexually abused as children, and women's responses to sexual violence by male intimates. She is the author of *Counseling Adult Survivors of Childhood Sexual Abuse.*

James J. Fletcher received his B.A. from Iona College, New Rochelle, New York; his M.A. from Marquette University, Milwaukee; and his Ph.D. from Indiana University, Bloomington. He is an associate professor of philosophy in the Department of Philosophy and Religious Studies at George Mason University in Fairfax, Virginia. He has been a member of the George Mason faculty since 1972, serving in a variety of teaching and administrative capacities, includ-

253

ing 15 years in the office of the provost. He teaches courses in ethics, bioethics, and philosophy of technology. His current research interests in bioethics include organizational ethics for healthcare providers and end-of-life issues. In addition, he has written and presented extensively on higher education issues relating to instruction and to faculty roles and rewards. He is the ethics collaborator in the Office of Health Care Ethics in the College of Nursing and Health Science at George Mason. He is the chair of one institutional review board and member of another. Dr. Fletcher serves as a community member of the Prince William Health Systems Bioethics Committee, for which he provides consultancies and educational programming.

Joanne M. Hessmiller, M.S.W., Ph.D., is a member of the faculty of the Graduate School of Social Work at Marywood University in Scranton, Pennsylvania. Active in the battered women's movement since 1982, her primary focus of practice and main research interest has been the prevention of intimate violence. She is the educational supervisor for the ADVANCE program of Lutheran Social Services (a batterer intervention program in York, Pennsylvania), and she provides training and consultation in batterer intervention program development, violence prevention, trauma, and critical incident stress and nonviolent conflict resolution for schools and organizations. Dr. Hessmiller is one of the collaborative authors of *Accountability: Program Standards for Batterer Intervention Programs.*

Pamela M. Ironside, Ph.D., R.N., is an associate professor in the Department of Nursing and Health at Clarke College in Dubuque, Iowa. She teaches research design, research seminar, nursing theories, perspectives on nursing, and a variety of nursing education courses including curriculum development, instruction, and clinical education. Her current research uses interpretive phenomenology to explicate the lived experiences of teachers, students, and citizens in nursing education toward creating site-specific, community-driven pedagogies. She is also using a multimethod approach to evaluate narrative pedagogy—an alternative approach for nursing education—in introductory nursing courses. She has published research articles in *Journal of Advanced Nursing, Advances in Nursing Science,* and *Nursing and Health Care Perspectives.*

Kathryn Hopkins Kavanagh, Ph.D., is a visiting scholar at Towson University, Baltimore, and is a medical anthropologist and psychiatric–mental health clinical nurse specialist. Following 2 years as director of a baccalaureate nursing program on the Navajo and Hopi reservations, Dr. Kavanagh currently teaches cultural and medical anthropology in the University of Maryland system and is at work on a historical interpretation of the nurse training program at Sage Memorial Hospital in Ganado, Arizona, which from 1930 to 1950 was the only nursing program ever developed specifically for Native Americans. She developed and ran a summer field school for University of Maryland students with the Oglala Lakota people on the Pine Ridge Reservation in South Dakota. Widely published in cultural aspects of healthcare, she authored *Promoting Cultural Diversity: Strategies for Health Care Professionals* with Patricia Kennedy.

Carol Ann Rooks, a survivor with a sense of humor, was born in 1954 and was unwilling to be handicapped by diabetes, with which she lived from the age of eight. Dr. Rooks earned baccalaureate degrees in speech communication and in nursing, and an M.S. in critical care nursing. She practiced in medical centers in Chicago; New Brunswick, New Jersey; and Baltimore. With completion of a dissertation focused on culture and ethics in nursing—and speculating about what she would do if the transplant pager went off immediately prior to graduation—Dr. Rooks earned the Ph.D. in nursing at the University of Maryland, Baltimore, in 1995. Already employed as a nurse researcher at Mercy Hospital in Baltimore, she underwent transplantation there a few weeks later. Carol Ann Rooks died June 26, 1999.

Mary Cipriano Silva is a professor at George Mason University's College of Nursing and Health Science. She received her B.S.N. and M.S. from the Ohio State University and her Ph.D. from the University of Maryland, College Park. In addition, as a Kennedy Fellow in Medical Ethics for Nursing Faculty, she undertook postdoctoral study in healthcare ethics at Georgetown University. She also has been a visiting scholar at the Hastings Center, Garrison, New York. Dr. Silva is a professor and the director of the Office of Health Care Ethics at George Mason University. Her book, *Ethical Decision Making in Nursing Administration,* won an award from the *American Journal of Nursing,* and she has written extensively in the field of ethics. In 1995 she authored the American Nurses Association's (ANA) new guidelines on ethics in nursing research. In 1996 she was selected to be a member of the ANA Code of Ethics Project Task Force to revise the 1985 code. The newly revised Code of Ethics for Nurses was published in 2001. She is a member of the American Academy of Nursing's Expert Panel on Ethics. At present, she is engaged in research on administrative ethical issues in healthcare and on spirituality research.

Rebecca S. Sloan is assistant professor of nursing and past chair of the Qualitative Research Section of the Midwest Nursing Research Society. She received the Outstanding Researcher New Investigator award from the Chronicity Section of the Midwest Nursing Research Society in 2000. A nephrology nurse for more than 20 years, Dr. Sloan received her doctoral education in medical sociology, which contributes to her interdisciplinary approach to the concerns of persons experiencing chronic illness and their families. Her program of research in end-stage renal disease received national recognition with funding from the National Institute of Nursing Research and the NIH-sponsored Center for Excellence in Quality of Life in Chronic Illness in 2001.

Dr. Sloan uses interpretive phenomenology to explicate the meaning of living a life-sustained-by-medical-technology. Her current research program explores how patients readapt to dialysis a second time after loss of a kidney transplant.

Elizabeth Smythe is a principal lecturer at Auckland University of Technology, New Zealand. She teaches within an interdisciplinary masters of health science program and has a particular interest in midwifery knowledge and philosophical perspectives of practice. Her doctoral study explored the meaning of "being safe" in childbirth. She embraces the philosophical writings of Heidegger and Gadamer in her understandings of hermeneutic research. Dr. Smythe is active in international nursing and midwifery initiatives and is widely sought as a consultant in philosophy and practice.

Jeanne M. Sorrell received her B.S.N. from the University of Michigan–Ann Arbor, her M.S.N. from the University of Wisconsin–Madison, and her Ph.D. from George Mason University. She is a professor in the College of Nursing and Health Science at George Mason University, where she currently serves as coordinator of the Ph.D. in Nursing Program and coordinator of special projects in the Office of Health Care Ethics. Dr. Sorrell teaches graduate nursing courses on the scholarship of writing, research, education, and advanced clinical nursing. Her current research uses interpretive phenomenology to explore the lived experience of patients and caregivers with Alzheimer's Disease. Based on this research, she has produced an educational video, *Stories of Quality Lives: Ethics in the Care of Persons with Alzheimer's* to educate nurses and other healthcare professionals about important ethical considerations in the care of dementia patients.

Index

257